Dr At...
Age-De...

Diet Revolution

Also by Dr Robert C. Atkins

Dr Atkins New Diet Revolution
Dr Atkins New Diet Cookbook
Dr Atkins New Carbohydrate Counter

Dr Atkins
Age-Defying
Diet Revolution

Dr Robert C. Atkins
with Sheila Buff

Vermilion
LONDON

First published in 1992 by Vermilion
This edition published in 2003 by Vermilion
an imprint of Ebury Press, Random House,
20 Vauxhall Bridge Road, London SW1V 2SA
www.randomhouse.co.uk

Penguin Random House is committed to a sustainable future for
our business, our readers and our planet. This book is made from
Forest Stewardship Council® certified paper.

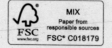

MIX
Paper from
responsible sources
FSC® C018179

Printed and bound in Great Britain by Clays Ltd, St Ives plc

A CIP catalogue record for this book is available from the British Library.

ISBN 978 0091887735

The advice offered in this book, although based on the
author's experience with many thousands of patients, is not
intended to be a substitute or the advice and counsel of your
personal physician. Always consult a medical practitioner
before embarking on a diet. Neither the Author nor the
Publisher can be held responsible for any loss or claim arising
out of the use, or misuse, of the suggestions made, or the
failure to take medical advice.

To my many activist followers,
who are determined to spread
the truths that will make
the world a healthier place

CONTENTS

PART III

AGE-DEFYING NUTRIENTS

PART IV

TECHNIQUES TO DEFY AGING

PART V

LIVING THE AGE-DEFYING DIET

Contents

NOTE TO THE READER

The information offered in this book, although based on the author's experience with many thousands of patients, is not intended to be a substitute for the advice and counsel of your personal physician. While the recommendations are appropriate for most people, each individual may have different requirements based on a full medical profile. No one regime fits all.

PREFACE

This is not the first book ever written on the subject of anti-aging or longevity medicine or rejuvenation. Just about every health writer seems to be taking a crack at it nowadays. But if you're the least bit familiar with me, you know I won't be coming to the same conclusions or recommending the same strategies as others have done.

That's because I write from a unique vantage point—I've been a full-time medical practitioner for more than forty years. In that time, The Atkins Center in New York City has treated and impacted the lives of more than sixty-five thousand people who have come to us as patients. The vast majority have accomplished what this book promises. They have become younger—not chronologically, since no one can turn back time—but by all the usual medical measures. This means that their physical, mental, and laboratory findings remain better than they were when they first came to us, and/or the rate at which they showed the problems attributed to aging were slowed down, often to a remarkable degree.

I am one of those people whose purpose in life has always been to be "a seeker of truth." As a physician, the truth I was seeking was whatever would work best to help my patients overcome their illnesses. My career, in large part, was shaped by a lesson I learned after my first book was written. That lesson was that what doctors are taught is "the truth" is all too often anything but.

My solution was to rely on my own experience and to draw my own conclusions from that. I learned to accept no dogmatic pronouncements or judgments from the consensus of medical leaders unless they were confirmed by my own experience. This stubbornly independent pursuit of the truth led to my success as a physician, teacher, and author.

But as I became more well-known and received acclaim from my followers and venom from my critics, I never ceased being a seeker. Therefore I never allowed myself to lose sight of the other pathway by which I sought knowledge—from the teachings of my colleagues in the scientific community.

Well, in the past decade or two, these scientists have made an incredible series of discoveries. I have tried many of their exciting breakthroughs on my patients—and on myself—and have confirmed that certain of them work very well.

And so I am in a position to share with you the techniques that are proving to be most promising for my patients in their quest to look and feel younger, healthier, stronger, more vigorous, and more mentally alert. I believe that the techniques that work now will prove to have lasting value, giving those who follow them a longer life with all the virtues preserved.

Let's see how we will do it.

Part I tells you why you too must learn to defy conventional wisdom in order to defy age. Part II explains the causes of aging. Here's what you'll learn:

- Many of the seemingly inevitable diseases of aging—heart disease, osteoporosis, senility, failing eyesight, and more—are not inevitable at all. They can be easily prevented or ameliorated by avoiding the causes of aging.
- What makes us age? In large part, it's what we eat. In the westernized world we eat far too much sugar, refined

carbohydrates, and processed fats. These foods cause blood sugar disorders and obesity—the first steps down the slippery slope to heart disease, kidney disease, and a host of other life-shortening ailments.

- The typical American diet is a recipe for the one thing that will age you faster than anything: high blood sugar and the elevated insulin levels that invariably accompany it.

- A low-carbohydrate, high-protein diet is the single most effective way to lose weight and to normalize your blood sugar.

- Most researchers today agree that the underlying cause of aging, especially the accelerated aging that flows from the Western diet, is accumulated damage to our bodies from free radicals. (This is such a crucial concept that I devote all of Chapter 6 to it.)

Once I've explained the major causes of aging, I move on in Part III to discuss antioxidants—the age-defying foods, vitamins, minerals, and other supplements that prevent or block damage from free radicals.

- Antioxidants in the diet come primarily from fresh vegetables and fruits and unrefined carbohydrates. A diet high in sugar and refined carbohydrates has little room for these foods.

- To defy age, we must also use a range of safe, highly effective antioxidant supplements.

The age-defying techniques I use at the Atkins Center start with diet but go far beyond it. Among the techniques I'll discuss in Part IV are:

- Hormone optimizing to restore your hormones to more youthful levels—a subject so important that I have devoted two long chapters to it.
- Improving your immunity through dietary change and vitanutrients (nutrients vital to good health) such as vitamin A, zinc, and garlic.
- Detoxifying your body through chelation therapy and by restoring your intestinal tract to a desirable balance.
- Exercising for a healthier heart, better glucose tolerance, lower blood pressure, and weight loss.
- Boosting your brain power with vitanutrients such as ginkgo biloba.

In Part V, I detail the heart of this book: how to live the age-defying diet. Here you'll learn the basics of the diet:

- How to defy conventional wisdom and ignore the "food pyramid."
- How to select low-carbohydrate, nutrient-dense foods that stabilize your blood sugar and are also rich sources of antioxidants.
- How to choose the right fats and avoid the dangerous ones.
- How to tailor the diet to your individual needs and discover the carbohydrate intake level that is best for you.
- How to decide which supplements you need to take, and in what amounts.

We've got a lot of territory to cover—and you're getting older by the minute. It's time to get started.

PART I

An Introduction to Defying Aging

In this part, I'll introduce my convention-defying ideas about aging. You'll learn:

▬

That many of the common diseases of aging can be prevented or reduced through proper diet and vitanutrients.

▬

What's wrong with the diet-heart hypothesis.

▬

Why the low-fat diet recommended by conventional medicine is the diet you should never follow.

▬

How to lower your cholesterol the natural way, without dangerous drugs.

1

Defiance and Dietary Know-How: The Keys to Holding Back Aging

The first words I wrote for this book were its title. The subject was a foregone conclusion; now that I'm approaching seventy, it's difficult to focus on any subject other than making sure that I stay eternally young. That focus has led to enough productive experience that I'm sure I can pass on some pretty exciting information to you.

Whenever I reflect on what I must teach you to age-proof yourself, as much as can be, the word "defiance" always jumps into my consciousness. This relates less to defying the aging process, as the title of this book would lead you to believe, than to *defying the prevailing beliefs*. The more I learn about how to live more and more years without feeling their effects, the more I realize that most of the information we are fed by the powers that be in the medical establishment is horribly misleading. I believe it is so misleading as to be responsible for most of the avoidable physical and mental decline that we interpret as aging.

So lesson number one will be: To defy aging, you must first learn to defy what the authorities are trying to teach you. Don't think I won't elaborate on this point; I absolutely must do so. Too many of you are diligently following rules of good health that seem so well accepted that you assume they are established facts, such as eating a low-fat diet and eating lots of grains and fruits. Unfortunately, the dishonest side of the dogma presented to you may be the very obstacle that is holding you back from achieving your goal of a long and healthy life.

The title's fourth word, "diet," is a bit of poetic license. I've developed a reputation for providing rather effective diets, and this may cause some people to lose sight of the value of all of the nutritional approaches we use. This book will not focus on showing you how to lose weight the luxurious Atkins way, although it will certainly help you do so if you need to. So, hereinafter, let's understand that "Age-Defying Diet" refers to an overall age-defying nutritional plan.

The title's fifth word, "revolution," is one I'm sure you'll recognize and associate with my approach to nutrition and health. It defines what I've been trying to accomplish with my life's work—to make the populace so aware of the economic self-interest behind the medical establishment, and its efforts to get us to succumb to its profit-based dogma, that we silently revolt against it.

The twentieth century's impact on health can be defined as the conflict between scientists who make discoveries and scientists who make policy. The result is that much more of what you need to defy aging is known than you are being told. The current of scientific discovery provides the information we need to achieve our goals, but the current of economic self-interest preserves the status quo and prevents those break-throughs from getting the widespread use and acceptance they deserve.

All of us will be better served if this new millennium begins with the rejection of those whose interests are not consonant with those of the general public and the acceptance of those who are determined to lead us out of the morass the medical mainstream has created.

The many favorable experiences achieved by Atkins Center patients have helped me determine how to present you with the best techniques for reversing the aging process. I will teach you all the basic programs we have developed to get our patients healthier.

You'll learn why we age and how we can slow the process. You'll learn specific ways to optimize your nutrition, idealize your hormone levels, rejuvenate aging organs, remove accumulations of toxins, restore healthy bacteria to your digestive tract, avoid adverse environmental elements, optimize your brain nutrition, and much more.

Throughout, I'll emphasize that most of what we call aging is simply the presence of disease—chronic, seemingly ubiquitous disease that makes us age with such apparent time-dependent consistency that we accept it universally as "simply getting older." Nothing could be farther from the truth. Many of the common ailments of aging can be prevented or reduced through proper diet and supplemental vitanutrients—my overall term for vitamins, minerals, herbs, and other supplements.

No one yet seems to have noticed that getting old today is quite different from a hundred years ago. The irony is that coronary heart disease, the major illness associated with age, was virtually unheard of a century ago. If we could eradicate atherosclerotic cardiovascular disease, the major disease of the twentieth—and now the twenty-first—century, we would extend our life span by easily four to six years or even a dozen years. They would be healthy years, unmarred by chronic illness and disability. Heart disease *can* be eradicated, and therefore, that's where I'd like to begin defying aging.

Learn to Separate Fact from Fiction

It should take very little convincing for you to accept the idea that eliminating cardiovascular disease would be a very effective first step in extending our collective life spans. You know full well that heart disease kills more of us than any other condition, and that narrowed, poorly functioning blood vessels cause even more of us to show signs of aging and limit our ability to enjoy our lives. Every organ, every part of your body, from your brain to the bottoms of your feet, ages when it no longer gets a good supply of blood.

But I'll wager it will take some major convincing to bring you to the same conclusion reached decades ago, which has allowed me to reverse the time clock on thousands of my patients. That simple conclusion is that people have been lied to about heart disease with such an intense barrage of misinformation for so long that even honest scholarly researchers are repeating these whoppers without a smidgen of suspicion that they could be untrue.

It is clear, then, that even before we learn how heart disease can be slowed down and actually reversed, we must learn the truth about what seems to be the conventional wisdom.

I'm sure we're all familiar with "the Gospel According to the American Heart Association." It's the same advice adopted by the American Medical Association, American Dietetic Association, the U.S. government, and the National Cholesterol Education Program (NCEP). All of them seem to agree unquestioningly that:

- All dietary fats must be restricted, especially saturated ones.
- Dietary cholesterol must be nearly eliminated.
- Margarine and other polyunsaturated fats are more healthful than butter and other saturated fats.
- Carbohydrates made with white flour should be the basis of a healthful diet.
- Eating ten teaspoons of sugar a day is perfectly good for you.

New scientific information from even the most prestigious journals that points clearly to the deleterious effects of trans fats (dangerous fats found in processed fats such as margarine) and refined junk carbohydrates made with sugar and white flour is clearly not heeded by the medical establishment. This is nowhere so well illustrated as in the American Heart Association's "Heart-Check" seal of approval on high-sugar, empty-calorie foods. You can see the Heart-Check symbol on all sorts of worthless foods, including breakfast cereals. These foods are often nothing but refined carbohydrates and may be as much as 50 percent sugar—but they have less than 3 grams of fat per serving. The AHA's unmistakable message: "Avoid fats, and nothing else matters."

Despite the obvious errors of judgment displayed by the spokespeople for the medical establishment, the overwhelming majority of nutritionally concerned citizens stand by the low-fat guidelines, secure in the knowledge that forty years of scientific studies have proved this point beyond any doubt.

But have they? Here's a major take-home message from this book: *Nothing could be farther from the truth.* The billions of research dollars (much of it from your taxes in the form of government-sponsored work) spent to support the hypothesis that dietary fat leads to heart disease have, with remarkable consistency, proved the strategy to be a failure.

Let's look at the facts and you'll see for yourself. Of the dozens of proven items that call the imaginary diet-heart hypothesis into question, none is more straightforward than the well-documented truth that heart attacks (myocardial infarction) were so rare at the start of the twentieth century that the first case was not described until 1912. In 1930, heart attacks caused no more than three thousand deaths in the United States.[1]

Based on this figure, it behooves us to ask what Americans

were consuming in the early part of the century. The amount of fat in the average daily diet then was somewhat greater than it is today, when we are in the midst of an epidemic of heart attacks. The fat we ate in 1900 was mainly butter, lard, and tallow (beef fat). Don't these facts demand an explanation? The AHA don't give one so I guess it's up to me to explain why today's official dietary recommendations could be dangerous to your health. Let's start with a closer look at the history of the diet-heart hypothesis.

Diet and Your Heart: A Brief History

Ancel Keys was the famed nutritional researcher selected to determine the nutritional needs of GIs and design portable meals to meet those needs. He's the "K" in K rations. (Whether he was also responsible for the decision to include a cigarette with every K ration pack, I couldn't say.)

With World War II over, however, Keys turned his attention to a review of diet and health around the world. The results of his Seven Countries study, revealed in the early 1950s, supposedly showed that people in countries where the typical diet was high in saturated fat had higher rates of heart disease. Unfortunately, Keys's reputation and standing were so great that the medical establishment immediately embraced his conclusions.

Based on the Keys Seven Countries study and others, equally flawed, the AHA undertook a campaign to replace butter, lard, eggs, and beef with corn oil, margarine, and cereal. By 1956, the campaign was in full swing. "Beware saturated fats" was the party line, and the medical establishment fell into place reciting it—with one notable exception. Dr. Paul Dudley White, Harvard's leading cardiologist (and President Dwight Eisenhower's physician), pointed out that he hadn't seen a single coronary at Harvard beween 1921 and 1928. On a televised panel discussion with other leading physicians he said, "Back in the myocardial-infarction-free days before 1920, the fats were butter and lard and I think we would all benefit from that kind of diet." His sensible advice, based on years of clinical experience and not epidemiological studies, was ignored.

A decade later, there was still no real proof of the diet-heart hypothesis. That didn't stop a manufacturer of corn oil and margarine from distributing a book in which Dr. Jeremiah Stamler affirmed that the theory was "enough to call for altering some habits even before the final proof is nailed down." In an effort to find that proof, Dr. Norman Jolliffe developed what he called the Prudent Diet, recruiting a bunch of middle-aged businessmen to try it. The diet emphasized corn oil, margarine, and cereal. The control group stuck to eggs, butter, and meat. The results? There were eight deaths from heart disease in the Prudent group versus none in the meat-and-potatoes group.

Even so, the diet-heart hypothesis was already so firmly entrenched that it couldn't be uprooted. Agribusiness had far too much invested in vegetable oils, corn, wheat, and highly profitable processed foods to allow any opposition—and it had the money and government clout to bulldoze its opponents. The food industry combined with the medical establishment in strenuous efforts to suppress dissenting opinions from such eminent scientists as Dr. Fred Kummerow of the University of Illinois, nutritional scientist Dr. Mary Enig, and Dr. George V. Mann of Vanderbilt University. Insiders have told me that what I considered to be an inappropriate attack on my low-carbohydrate diet by the American Medical Association in 1973 was engineered by the selfsame corn, vegetable oil, and cereal interests.

According to the early results of the ongoing Framingham

Heart Study, those with higher total cholesterol levels had slightly more "heart events." As I'll explain later, the connection between saturated fat in the diet and high total cholesterol was never really made. In fact, in 1992 the study's original director, Dr William Castelli, revealed the inside story on Framingham, pointing out that the people with lowest serum cholesterol were the ones who ate the most saturated fat and cholesterol and took in the most calories.[2]

With billions of dollars being invested to prove that cereal, corn oil, and margarine were heart-healthy and that most of us were candidates for cholesterol-lowering drugs, dozens of major international studies were conducted and published, all designed to ensure that the diet-heart hypothesis gained acceptance.

And gain acceptance it did—so well that it is still widely accepted today. The drop in death rates from cardiovascular disease between 1950 and 2000 is often cited in support of limiting fat in the diet. The overall decrease in the number of coronary episodes[3] over the past fifty years is wonderful news, but there is just one glaring shortcoming from the diet-heart point of view: Almost all of the decrease can be attributed to the significant decline in cigarette smoking (42 percent of all adults smoked in 1970, compared to less than 30 percent in 1996), better control of blood pressure, and improved treatments for heart attack. Putting the nation on a low-fat diet—an effort that has been notably unsuccessful—has had very little to do with our declining death rate from heart attacks. Heart disease is still the leading cause of death in the U.S.—it killed some 727,000 people in 1997. Today you're more likely to survive a heart attack, but your chance of still being alive five years later have hardly budged over the past twenty years. Some 24 percent of men and 42 percent of women will die within one year of having a myocardial infarction; within six years of a first heart attack, 21 percent of men and 33 percent of women will have another, 7 percent of men and women will experience sudden death, and 21 percent of the men and 30 percent of the women will be disabled with heart failure.[4] And even with the declining death rate from heart attacks, your lifetime risk of developing heart disease is still one in two for men and one in three for women.[5]

Now that the death rate from heart attacks is coming down, we're experiencing an epidemic of heart failure instead, because a myocardial infarction damages and weakens your heart, causing it gradually to stop working efficiently. The number of heart failure patients nearly doubled in the ten years from 1989 to 1999.[6] In many cases, heart failure is simply the delayed result of having a heart attack and being treated by conventional doctors with cholesterol-lowering statin drugs. These drugs block your ability to produce coenzyme Q_{10}, which is essential for producing energy in your cells, especially your heart cells. A shortage of CoQ_{10} is almost certain to make a weakened heart get weaker and fail, as I'll discuss in great detail in Chapter 9.

I've spent a good deal of time and effort to instill in you a critical attitude to the prevailing teachings about heart disease, because I soon will be telling you how the doctors and patients at the Atkins Center reverse this most important age-inducing disorder. But before I leave this subject, I feel I must show you how profoundly the prevailing teachings can adversely affect every aspect of your health.

The number-one unifier between the American Heart Association, American Medical Association, American Diabetes Association, and U.S. government in its many manifestations (FDA, Department of Agriculture, NIH, et al.) is clear: All these organizations have gotten squarely behind the belief that "one diet fits all."

Now, I appreciate that you are not an academic in health science, but I am confident you are a person of extreme common sense. So let me direct this question to you for your commonsense answer. Do you believe that each and every one of us should be following the selfsame diet? Do you believe that fat people and thin ones, young and old, diabetics and heart patients, Jack Sprat and his wife, should all be eating exactly the same foods? Well, if it's as hard for you to accept as it is for me, then perhaps you are ready to see that the one-diet-fits-all belief is another fallacy to be rejected.

The second half of that fallacy is a direct cause of more premature aging than the first: ". . . and that one-fits-all diet contains all the nutrients anyone needs." Vitanutrients are part of the first line of defense against aging and age-mimicking illness. Suppressing them can adversely affect health. Throughout this book, I will discuss the exciting, well-documented, and easy-to-do aspects of defying aging through nutritional measures. In Chapter 22, I will present you with a summary of the Atkins Center protocols, with dosage ranges and more. Whether or not specifically mentioned in connection with each recommendation, please remember that everyone is a little—or maybe a lot—different and that you must take into account your full medical profile, with the assistance of your physician, before embarking on your age-defying regime.

I'm here to reawaken the seeds of doubt in your collective consciousness. Maybe now you will see why I say that defying aging begins with defying the conventional misteachings. To understand how you too can learn to defy aging, you'll first need to understand why we age at all. That's what I'll explain in Part II.

PART II

Why We Age

Must we just accept that with aging inevitably comes disease? No! In this part I'll explain why.

▬

Many of the seemingly inevitable diseases of aging—heart disease, osteoporosis, senility, failing eyesight, and more—can easily be prevented or ameliorated by avoiding the causes of aging.

▬

What makes us age? I'll discuss some leading theories and focus on the one theory that many researchers, myself included, believe is the true cause of aging: damage from free radicals.

▬

The typical American diet—high in sugar, refined carbohydrates, and processed fats—is a recipe for the one thing that will age you faster than anything else: blood sugar disorders.

2

The Diseases of Westernization

To many, the twentieth century was a major disappoint-
ment to those who were hoping for significant breakthroughs in overcoming aging. That is because, as the
nineteenth century's life-shortening illnesses were conquered,
new illnesses came along to keep us decades from our goal.
Heart disease, diabetes, hypertension, cancer, Alzheimer's disease, and other maladies for all intents and purposes origi-
nated, or at least achieved epidemic proportions, in the
twentieth century—and they're getting more widespread in the
twenty-first. Objective observers have every right to say, "We
made progress in overcoming infectious disease and conditions that strike us down in our youth, but the older ones
among us still reach senility at approximately the same age."

I see it differently. The twentieth century ended with the
scientific know-how to eradicate the very illnesses that defined
that century. The political and economic know-how may still
elude us, but the scientific avant garde have done their job and
the fruits of their collective labor are available to us now.

Eradicate the quintessential twentieth-century ailment—

atherosclerotic cardiovascular disease—and we will, scientists have estimated, extend our collective life expectancy by twelve years. We started the century with a collective life expectancy of forty-five years and, at last count, had expanded it to 76.5 years on average.[1] With the intelligent eradication of atherosclerotic heart disease we have the know-how quickly to reach ninety. Before 1900, 75 percent of all Americans died before age sixty-five; today, more than 70 percent of us will live to be over seventy. Improving human life expectancy so profoundly in a single century does not make that century a failure.

I hope I just said something that got your attention. Heart disease, the illness that caused the premature death of most of us just a couple of generations ago, was virtually unheard of seventy-five years ago!

Imagine that, starting now, we could begin to reduce the incidence of heart disease, diabetes, stroke, and hypertension. What would all these changes do for our life expectancy? If we could eliminate heart disease, now the number-one cause of mortality in the industrialized world, we would gain an estimated twelve years or more of life expectancy—and, of course, avoid the years of ill health that heart disease can cause before it kills you. We've made a good start on this—had heart disease continued at the same rate as its peak in 1963, 621,000 additional people would have died from it.[2] And if we could eliminate diabetes, stroke, and hypertension, all major contributors to causes of death other than heart disease, the gain in life expectancy would be even greater.

Those of you who know me from my previous writings, lectures, and broadcasts will recognize that the illnesses singled out by health history as twentieth-century diseases are the ones to which I have given the name "diet-related disorders." The term was not given casually, to indicate that it just seems as if diet plays a role in their cause. Rather, the term reflects a conclusion that became inescapable when I revamped the diet and vitanutrient intake of my patients and saw their illnesses dramatically reverse themselves and often go away entirely.

It is no coincidence that the majority of illnesses that distinguish today's "killer diseases" are diet-related disorders. This whole book, like all my books, is designed to explain why that is and help you avoid these diseases yourself by modifying your own diet. Now I would like to share with you a major piece of scientific evidence in the diet-related disorder puzzle. It is evidence that has deeply influenced my own work.

Dr. Cleave and the Rule of Twenty Years

In 1974, a brilliant physician named T. L. Cleave, a surgeon-captain in the Royal Navy and a former director of medical research at the Institute of Naval Medicine, published an epidemiological study called *The Saccharine Disease*. This work, now unfortunately out of print, has long had my vote for the number-one health book of the twentieth century.

Cleave made a careful study of hospital records of third world nations, mainly in Africa, and he was struck that virtually no single native came down with the common diseases of Western cultures such as obesity, diabetes, colon cancer, gallstones, diverticulitis, and heart disease. The common Western illnesses were not simply less frequent; they were nonexistent.

Unlike his colleague Dr. Dennis Burkitt, who looked at the same type of data and concluded that the high dietary fiber these people ate was what protected them, Cleave was convinced that it was the other side of the coin that did the trick. The absence of refined carbohydrates in the diets protected against twentieth-century illness. Cleave painstakingly demonstrated that almost exactly twenty years after introducing

Western foods to the diet and letting them replace the native foods, diabetes and heart disease would begin to appear in the population. Within forty years, these diseases would be widespread. Cleave dubbed this his Rule of Twenty Years, and I've seen it proved time and again.

One particular piece of evidence clinched Cleave's explanations for me. Studies in Israel showed that twenty years after Yemenite Jews moved to Israel and gave up their traditional diet of unrefined, natural foods in favor of a more westernized diet that was high in sugar and other refined carbohydrates, diabetes began to appear. Diabetes was basically unknown among these people while they still lived a traditional life in Yemen. In fact, they were thought to be genetically free of the disease.

Cleave observed that roughly twenty years after a society introduces refined carbohydrates to its way of life, diabetes and heart disease will simultaneously begin to appear. The Yemenites proved to be a perfect case in point. In 1977, about twenty-five years after they had immigrated to Israel, their rate of diabetes and glucose intolerance was 11.8 percent, quite similar to the rest of community.[3] Cleave cited a number of similar examples, particularly among Icelanders and Pacific Islanders.

More recently, Cleave's Rule of Twenty Years has been borne out in other studies. The Pima Indians of Arizona have such a high rate of kidney failure from diabetes that their reservation has its own dialysis center. In Saudi Arabia, diabetes and associated heart disease have emerged almost exactly twenty years after refined carbohydrates and a more westernized diet became the norm. Today in Saudi Arabia, diabetes afflicts 12 percent of the men and 14 percent of the women who live in urban areas. Among urban women age fifty-one to sixty, the prevalence of diabetes is an astonishing 49 percent. In the rural populations, where people still have some remnants of their traditional diet, the rates are lower but still high: 7 percent for men and 7.7 percent for women. Saudi Arabia has gone from being a country that had virtually no diabetes before 1970 to having one of the highest rates of diabetes in the world.[4]

Cleave's Rule of Twenty Years is also proving true in Japan, India, Mexico, and many other countries. His hypothesis of the linkage of refined carbohydrates to both diabetes and atherosclerosis has been proved beyond any reasonable doubt.

Cleave's discoveries have never been refuted; indeed, they have proved prophetic. Cleave's Rule of Twenty Years taught us when the very first cases of diabetes-induced heart disease would appear, but its greatest value, in my opinion, lies in predicting when epidemic increases in these conditions will take place in cultures varied enough already to have some familiarity with these conditions.

The Diet Distinction

By applying the Rule, these questions can now be readily answered: Why were cardiologists a minor specialty in Japan in the 1950s yet are a major necessity now? Why is Asia the new hotbed of a diabetes epidemic exceeding 100 million cases? Why does the World Health Organization project a 170 percent growth in the number of people with diabetes in developing countries by 2025, from 84 million to 228 million people? Why is the worldwide rise projected to be 122 percent, from 135 million to 300 million people? Why will diabetes nearly double in India between 1995 and 2025?[5]

The answer to all these questions is the same: They are the consequence of the westernization of these cultures, which in biologic terms means the dietary acceptance of refined carbohydrates. Thus, Cleave's discoveries provide a large part of the basis for understanding the incidence of modern illness in all parts of the world.

Cleave's *Saccharine Disease* may have been an observation noted before its time, referring to the fact that the phenomenon was observed before the scientific explanation was worked out. But all that is water under the bridge. So much evidence has been amassed linking refined carbohydrates to sugar and insulin disorders, and these disorders to heart disease, hypertension, and stroke, that any medical advisory board member entrusted with making public health policy should not overlook it, and it raises concerns about the American Heart Association continuing to recommend sugar-laden cereals.

Important scientific journals now abound with information about risk factors for heart disease, and it is becoming increasingly apparent that the total cholesterol level is relatively minor when compared to other biochemical abnormalities much more likely to lead to our number-one cause of death and of shortened life span. I do not believe there is a practicing cardiologist who is unaware of these facts, but it is quite possible that, if you consult one, you may not hear of them.

Fixed ideas are hard to dislodge. So in the next few chapters, I will lay out these facts for you, based on the knowledge available now. There's no better target for our exploration than our number-one killer—heart disease.

3

Aging, Carbohydrates,
and Your Heart

Protect Those Blood Vessels!

I am quite enamored of the many recent scientific breakthroughs that give us reason for optimism about holding
back the aging process. Nonetheless, I think for now we must
maintain our focus on the one illness most capable of causing
us to age prematurely: cardiovascular disease, officially known
as atherosclerosis.

The most dramatic way it ends our lives is by a fatal heart
attack (myocardial infarction), a blockage of one or more of the
major arteries that supply blood to our hearts. A heart attack is
the culmination of a long process of heart disease that starts
many years earlier. The process involves the blocking of other
arteries that feed your heart and other organs. The decline in
blood circulation and therefore organ function caused by the
blockage is considered by conventional medicine to be a "normal" part of the process of aging when it takes place in an older
person.

Do you really believe that? You know from Chapter 2 that

atherosclerosis hasn't been around all that long—it's become common only over the past century. People have been aging for a lot longer than that. Given enough time, everyone ages, but not everyone gets heart disease. Clearly, there's nothing "normal" about atherosclerosis at all.

That's exactly why fighting off atherosclerosis presents the window of greatest opportunity to make real inroads in reversing the aging process. All we have to do is wipe out an illness that very few humans even got until four generations ago.

What Causes Heart Disease?

The evidence clearly demonstrates that there is no single cause of heart disease. Quite reasonably, then, no single program can prevent it. The best you can do is discover what might make you uniquely vulnerable to heart problems, based on your own personal risk factors.

To start with, that means getting a complete evaluation of your blood to include all possible risk factors for heart disease. Lab test results by themselves are useless, however; you must have them analyzed by a doctor who recognizes that there are many paths to heart disease.

Far too many physicians still look at only your cholesterol figures and don't bother to test for anything else. That can be very misleading.

Your total cholesterol figure is essentially the sum of two figures: one good, the high-density or HDL cholesterol, and one bad, the low-density or LDL cholesterol. You want the HDL to be as high as possible and the LDL to be as low as possible. So it isn't the total number that counts; it's the ratio. You can be sure that a football fan will be much happier with a game in which 91 total points are scored and his team wins 49–42 than one in which only 10 points are scored and his favorites lose 7–3.

A complete blood evaluation, therefore, should start with a full lipid profile, looking at the amounts of different kinds of fats in your blood—not just LDL and HOL cholesterol but triglycerides (TG), very low-density lipoproteins (VLDL), and lipoprotein(a), abbreviated as Lp(a), as well. Each of these lipid profile measures tells us something different—and each tells us something important.

Understanding Your Lipid Profile

Let's start with some definitions. Cholesterol is a waxy fat your body needs for many crucial functions, such as making hormones, cell walls, and nerve sheaths. About 85 percent of the cholesterol in your body is made in your liver and in the cells of your small intestine; the rest comes from your diet.

Cholesterol is waxy, which means it's not soluble in water. To carry cholesterol around in your bloodstream, which is mostly water, your body coats it with protein—that's why we call the various types of fatty particles floating in your blood lipoproteins (from the Greek *lipos*, meaning "fat"). The more protein a cholesterol particle carries, the denser it is. About 65 percent of the circulating lipoprotein in your blood is low-density lipoprotein. LDLs carry cholesterol to your cells. About 20 percent of your circulating lipoproteins is high-density lipoprotein, or HDL cholesterol. These smaller, denser cholesterol particles are "good" because they pick up cholesterol from your cells and carry it back to the liver for further processing.

Triglycerides are very small, light fat particles. Your body sends some of your triglycerides to your muscles for energy and stores some as body fat. Triglycerides are converted in the liver into very low-density lipoproteins. VLDL may well be the unsung villain of the blood lipids. Your VLDL level goes up along with your triglyceride level and may be just as danger-ous, in part because these particles get denser as they circulate in your blood.

HDL: The Good Cholesterol

For decades mainstream cardiologists have recognized the beneficial role played by the HDL cholesterol fraction. Every ratio indicating risk of heart disease uses it as the divisor. Be it the total cholesterol, the LDL, the LDL plus VLDL, or the dramatically important triglycerides, all are divided by the HDL—and all these numbers, when they rise, will cause your doctor great concern. Conclusion: HDL is one number you want to be as high as possible.

How can you get it high and keep it there? Not with a low-fat diet—quite the contrary. HDL is *lowered* by a low-fat diet, not so much by the absence of fat but by the increased con-sumption of carbohydrates that accompanies fat restriction.

What About the Bad Cholesterol?

I presume by now you're asking, "If the whole world says cho-lesterol is bad, why are you saying it's good?" Well, I'm not really saying that—I've just singled out the HDL for the honor. High total cholesterol is problematic only if it is high because of high LDL *and* low HDL. Indeed, LDL ("bad" cholesterol) is a bona fide risk factor—but only, as recent research demonstrates, when it is oxidized by free radicals. (I promise you, you'll be learning an awful lot about free radicals as you read on.)

Nonetheless, the heart risk created by oxidized LDL cholesterol is no greater than that created by the risk factors you'll be learning about—triglycerides, elevated homocysteine, lipoprotein(a), C-reactive protein, and others.

Cholesterol risk is overemphasized to the point where the other risk factors are too often ignored. Instead of looking at other risk factors, patients are being hustled into taking statin drugs, the darlings of the cholesterol-drug industry. I'll briefly state here that taking these drugs won't help you to live any longer. None of the first eighty major studies of cholesterol-lowering drugs demonstrated any significant extension of life span among patients using them. (Another recent study, one of the first done on a statin drug, reported an alarming paradox: Although there were considerably fewer heart attacks among those taking the drug, those who did have heart attacks while taking the drug had three times the death rate of the control group.)

Triglycerides

Today's tunnel vision fingering cholesterol as the sole cause of heart disease could mean that your doctor probably hasn't paid much attention to your triglyceride level, unless it's abnormally high.

You could pay for your doctor's ignorance with your life. Long ignored, high triglycerides have been convincingly shown to be an independent risk factor for heart disease. The higher your triglycerides, the greater your chance of a heart attack. If you're a woman, having high triglycerides is a particularly good predictor of heart disease. In other words, having high triglycerides is every bit as much of a risk factor for heart disease as is obesity, smoking, or high blood pressure.[2]

What makes triglycerides so dangerous? In large amounts, they thicken your blood and keep it from flowing easily through your blood vessels. When blood that should be watery turns sludgy from too many triglycerides, it clogs your blood vessels and forms clots. The result is often a blockage in the arteries feeding your heart—in short, you have a heart attack.

Most doctors believe the misinformation they were taught in medical school—that triglyceride levels of 250 to 500 mg/dl are perfectly normal. They're wrong, and their ignorance could kill you. Even 200 mg/dl is too high. As a matter of fact, you need to worry about your heart health when your triglycerides are anything above 100 mg/dl. If your level is above 100 mg/dl, you have twice the risk of suffering a fatal attack as someone whose level is in the 50- to 60-mg/dl range.[3]

High TG/Low HDL: A Deadly Combination

Having high triglycerides is bad enough, but even more deadly is the combination of high triglycerides and low HDL cholesterol. That dangerous duo dramatically raises your risk of a heart attack. Results from a multiyear study of men in Muenster, Germany, in the 1980s showed that only 4 percent had the combination, yet during the study period 25 percent of the heart attacks occurred among men in this group.[4]

It wasn't until 1997 that Dr. J. M. Gaziano and his colleagues at Harvard showed just how predictive of heart disease a high triglyceride/low HDL ratio really is. In this study, the participants were divided into four subgroups or quartiles according to ratios of triglycerides to HDL: highest, high middle, low middle, and lowest. The quartile with the highest ratio had sixteen times the likelihood of heart attacks as the lowest quartile.[5] The significance of such numbers is staggering. *No ratio has ever come close to being so predictive of heart disease.* If you are in the highest quartile, with, say, triglycerides of 190 and HDL of 37, having an ideal cholesterol of 180 still leaves you at great risk. But if your triglyceride level is no higher than your HDL, then having a total cholesterol of 300 may indicate very little heart risk.

It's pretty obvious, then, that your ratio of triglycerides to HDL cholesterol is critically important to your future heart health. Ideally, you want a ratio below 1:1, with your triglycerides lower than your HDL. Low triglycerides and high HDL mean a low likelihood of heart disease. If your ratio is 2:1, with your triglycerides higher than your HDL, you're on the borderline of normal. Anything higher than 2:1 is beginning to be serious, especially if you're over the 100 mg/dl mark for triglycerides. You're asking for heart trouble, trouble that simple dietary changes could help you avoid completely.

As I'll discuss later on in this book, a low-carbohydrate diet, combined with vitanutrients such as omega-3 fatty acids and vitamin C, can make high triglycerides plummet by 60 or even 80 percent in just a few weeks. I don't claim to have discovered this. It's been well-known, even if the conclusion is largely ignored, since the publication of a paper on the subject by P. K. Reissell's group at Harvard in 1966. The study demonstrated dramatic and consistent corrections of severely elevated triglyceride levels with a diet strikingly similar to the induction (very low carbohydrate) phase of the Atkins diet.[6]

Recently another very important reason for lowering your triglycerides has been discovered. Women with high triglyceride levels have a 70 percent higher risk for breast cancer than women with low levels. The high triglycerides seem to trigger a rise in levels of circulating estrogen, which is a significant risk factor for breast cancer.[7]

A surprising number of my patients have never had their triglyceride levels tested by their conventional physicians, but triglycerides can't be swept under the rug. Their importance is being recognized by an increasing body of evidence. One 1999 study showed that people with TG levels of 100 (previously thought to be quite a normal level) had twice the likelihood of a coronary event than people with levels of 50.[8] The inescapable conclusion: The lower you bring down your triglycerides, the less chance you'll have of getting cardiovascular disease. This applies more to women than to men; one study estimated that 75 percent of all heart attacks that women get are associated with elevated triglycerides.[9]

If you're a thoughtful reader, your next question may well be, "Why are triglyceride elevations so much more likely to lead to heart disease when they are combined with low levels of HDL than when they are not?" I can't give you an absolute answer. Theorists postulate that whatever causes triglyceride elevation will, if profound enough, interfere with the synthesis of HDL cholesterol. There is certainly no shortage of studies documenting the high insulin, high triglycerides, and low HDL cluster.

I have proved the answer to myself but have not yet tried to prove it scientifically. My proof lies in the more than thirty thousand before-and-after lipid profiles the Atkins Center has done on patients pre- and postcarbohydrate restriction. Most people with elevated triglycerides get a 60 to 80 percent drop in their TG, combined with a 15 to 30 percent increase in their HDL. My data are only retrospective and thus are of less scientific value than a controlled, double-blind study would be. Should the day come when someone replicates these findings (I have no doubt that any study will get the same results), this is what they will prove: *Both elevated triglycerides and low levels of HDL come from the overconsumption of refined carbohydrates and are correctable by the restriction of carbohydrates.*

Triglycerides and the Glycemic Index

Elevated triglycerides are a direct consequence of an excessive outpouring of insulin in response to eating an inordinate quantity of carbohydrates. (Triglycerides have long been known to rise and fall as our levels of insulin rise and fall.) The glycemic index is a standard scale used to measure the ability of carbohydrate-containing foods to elevate blood sugar and insulin levels, foods high on the scale are known to cause this glucose-insulin-triglyceride sequence. (See the appendix for a glycemic index chart.) High glycemic index foods are primarily refined or simple carbohydrates taken without protein or fat to buffer their response. A very significant 1999 study showed that carbohydrates that are high on the glycemic index are considerably worse than the rest for raising your TG level.[10]

On the glycemic index we use at the Atkins Center, white table sugar (glucose) is the standard food; it's given the scale number of 100. The lower the number, the lower the glycemic index of the food. Beans and lentils, for instance, are much lower on the scale than bread, sweets, and potatoes, but meat, eggs, fish, and fowl are virtually zero. That's why long-term Atkins dieters consistently develop higher HDL levels and lower TG levels.

Testing for Triglycerides

When you go for your triglyceride blood test, timing is very important. Unlike cholesterol, which isn't really affected by eating, your triglyceride level can jump sharply after you eat. Schedule your test for first thing in the morning, and don't eat anything or drink anything other than plain water for ten to twelve hours before.

Licking Lipoprotein(a)

Lipoprotein(a) is as good a leading predictor of heart disease as are high triglycerides. This is a blood fat to take very seriously. Lp(a) is actually a sticky protein that attaches to cholesterol. The molecules of Lp(a) attach to the LDL particles in your blood and give you a double whammy. Because they're so sticky, Lp(a) particles can cause blockages and clots in your arteries. Even worse, they can keep plasminogen, your body's natural clot-dissolving enzyme, from working properly. That means the clot could further damage your arteries or even cause a heart attack.

A blood test reveals your Lp(a) level. A reading of 20 mg/dl is normal. Anything between 20 and 30 mg/dl is borderline, and anything above 30 mg/dl is elevated.

If your Lp(a) is on the high side, you could be one of those unfortunate people who are genetically predisposed to high levels. It's more likely, though, that your elevated level is caused by what you eat. We know that one of the major causes of high lipoprotein(a) levels is eating large amounts of hydrogenated and partially hydrogenated fats—the dreaded trans fats I'll discuss at length in Chapter 14. We also know that a good way to lower your Lp(a) level is to eat more saturated fats. If you throw out the margarine and switch to butter, you're making a good start on lowering your lipoprotein(a) level.

You might be wondering why your body naturally makes something as potentially harmful as lipoprotein(a). What good does it do? That's a question the great chemist and two-time Nobel laureate Linus Pauling asked himself. His answer is very interesting. Humans and other primates, such as gorillas, are among the very few animals that can't make their own vitamin C (fruit-eating bats and guinea pigs are the others). Instead they have to get their vitamin C from the foods they eat. The same animals that can't make vitamin C are also the only ones to have lipoprotein(a) in their blood. Pauling, along with his colleague Dr. Mathias Rath, theorized that we have Lp(a) as a sort of fallback mechanism for times when we might have a shortage of vitamin C. That's because in normal amounts, Lp(a) works to keep your blood vessels strong, protect your arteries from damage, and help repair any damage that does occur—exactly the same thing that vitamin C does (among its many other crucial roles in your body).

To prove their theory, Pauling and Rath first caused atherosclerosis in guinea pigs and then kept them from getting any vitamin C. In the absence of vitamin C, the plaque accumulated lipoprotein(a). When the guinea pigs were given plenty of vitamin C, however, they didn't develop any plaque in their damaged arteries.[11]

What the Pauling-Rath theory suggests is that high levels of vitamin C—perhaps as high as several grams a day—keep lipoprotein(a) in check. They found that the amino acid lysine helped these patients considerably by rendering the lipoprotein(a) harmless, even without lowering the blood level.

The Pauling-Rath protocol, combined with a diet that's low in trans fats and high in saturated fats, and along with some other vitanutrients such as niacin and N-acetyl-cysteine, could either lower your lipoprotein(a) level or render it less trouble-some—all without medications.

Homocysteine: The Hidden Heart Harmer

Now that I've clarified the most important and prevalent heart risk, I'd like to turn to the most unnecessary one: elevated levels of an abnormal protein called homocysteine.

A normal by-product of metabolizing the amino acid me-thionine, homocysteine is usually cleared rapidly from your blood before it can damage your arteries. In some people, though, homocysteine levels become dangerously elevated. Most studies of the causes of heart disease seem to agree that about 10 percent of coronary deaths and a somewhat greater proportion of stroke deaths can be directly attributed to abnor-mally high levels of homocysteine. This translates to more than one hundred thousand deaths in the United States every year—many of them among people who had perfectly fine blood lipid levels and no other risk factors for heart disease.

More to the point, homocysteine may be one of the direct causes of aging itself. Australian researcher Michael Fenech, using the technique of measuring micronuclei in human lym-phocytes to determine damage to chromosomes (a well-accepted cause of aging), found that higher homocysteine levels resulted in more chromosomal damage.[12]

Homocysteine doesn't come from eating eggs or saturated fat; in fact, it doesn't come from what you eat at all. It's what you *don't* eat. Plain and simple, elevated homocysteine is a re-sult of vitamin deficiency. This major cause of cardiovascular aging comes from suboptimal blood levels of the B complex vitamins, especially folic acid, B_6, and/or B_{12}. You need these vitamins to make the enzymes that remove homocysteine efficiently from your body. When well-fed Americans still end up short on these absolutely crucial B vitamins, and when their doctors neglect to test for their homocysteine levels, it is the outrageous consequence of policy makers' refusal to accept scientifically demonstrated information.

For decades, the FDA has placed a stringent limitation on the amount of folic acid (folate), the single most important nutrient involved in homocysteine control, that could be legally permitted in a vitamin capsule. Even though numerous scientific studies have shown that folic acid is North America's number-one vitamin deficiency and is responsible not only for homocysteine's health-undermining capacity but for serious birth defects as well, the FDA is unmoved and won't lift the insupportable restrictions. To this day, folic acid is the only vitamin that carries any dosage limitation. Instead of removing this scientifically unjustifiable restriction, the FDA went for the "two wrongs make a right" theory. They ordered that the quintessential junk food—enriched white flour—be fortified with a tiny amount of folic acid. That means that in order to get more dietary folic acid, people will have to consume the food I often call the "scourge of the twentieth—and now twenty-first—century."

Dr. McCully and the Homocysteine Story

Here's the irony: Every single one of the deaths attributed to homocysteine elevations could have been easily prevented had those people been told to take folic acid supplements in sufficient amounts. Why weren't they? An explanation is very much in order.

The homocysteine risk was first called to the public's attention by Dr. Kilmer McCully in the late 1960s. He pointed out not only that this compound was causing fatal heart attacks from damaged blood vessels but also that it could always be normalized by taking adequate amounts of the B vitamins, especially folic acid plus B_6 and B_{12}.

Consider the impact of McCully's well-conducted research. Here was a major cause of heart deaths that would not sell corn oil, cereal, margarine, or drugs; it would sell vitamins.

However McCully saw his work branded as insignificant. It took fifteen years, during which time an estimated 1.5 million Americans died of homocysteine-related vascular disease, before numerous reports confirmed McCully's work and even found that levels of homocysteine previously considered normal were capable of tripling the incidence of heart disease. What we still don't know is exactly how homocysteine damages your arteries, but damage them it most certainly does.

Let's look at two recent studies that show just how important it is to keep your homocysteine level low. In 1997, a large multicenter European trial found that among men and women younger than age sixty, the overall risk of coronary and other vascular disease was 2.2 times higher in those with plasma homocysteine levels in the top fifth of the normal range, compared to those in the bottom four-fifths. The risk was independent of other factors, but it was notably higher in smokers and people with high blood pressure.[13]

Even mild elevated homocysteine levels increase your chances of death from any cause, not just heart disease. In a long-term study of nearly two thousand residents of western Jerusalem, the risk of death was twice as high among subjects with the highest levels of homocysteine as among those with the lowest levels. Subjects with a mildly to moderately elevated homocysteine levels had a 30 to 50 percent higher risk of death than those with lowest levels.[14]

Taking a properly dosed multivitamin with enough folic acid could virtually eliminate anyone's homocysteine-based problem. Yet the preaching of organizations such as the American Heart Association and an entire roster of similar groups has never wavered from their position that vitamins should come only from the food we eat and not be taken as supplements. To prove my point, here's the official American Heart Association recommendation on homocysteine: "Although evidence for the benefit of lowering homocysteine levels is lacking, patients at high risk should be strongly advised to follow an overall diet that ensures adequate intake of folic acid and vitamins B_6 and B_{12}."[15] Meanwhile, surveys in both the United States and Canada have fingered folic acid as the number-one vitamin deficiency.

The FDA has a fifty-year history of limiting the legal dosage of folic acid to 0.8 mg, an amount that is often not adequate to correct homocysteine elevations. This means that an individual savvy enough to take a daily multivitamin is unlikely to get enough folic acid to render homocysteine innocuous, because FDA regulations forbid putting in enough to make a difference. The specious rationale is that taking large doses of folic acid could mask a deficiency of vitamin B_{12}. The problem, if it is one, could easily be circumvented by simply testing for vitamin B_{12} deficiency before starting the folic acid. Hundreds of daily vitamin takers have come to me with elevated homocysteine levels, only to have them normalized when prescription-strength folic acid was given.

How to Make Your Homocysteine Perfect

Both the diagnosis and treatment of too much homocysteine are surprisingly simple and effective.

A homocysteine blood level is easily obtained. The risk is linear, meaning the higher the number, even in the "normal" range, the more urgent is the need to provide the necessary vitamins. Most people with readings of 8 μmol/L should take the supplements, and anyone whose reading is above 12 μmol/L absolutely must take them. (The original work in the 1980s indicated that readings up to 15 μmol/L were acceptable.)

The three vitamins involved are quite safe, and there is no reason not to take 100 mg of B_6, 2,000 mcg of B_{12}, and 10 mg of folic acid daily. In fact, *you must*. A recent study showed that a program with only 5 mg of folic acid and 500 mcg of B_{12} failed to reduce homocysteine levels in nearly one-third of the patients in the trial.[16]

C-Reactive Protein: A New Marker of Heart Disease

Following a healthful diet is indeed a major answer to our current high levels of preventable heart disease, but unfortunately for some people, it is not the only answer. Some heart patients have very few of the usual risk factors, such as high triglycerides or obesity, for heart disease. One thing they do have, however, is high levels of C-reactive protein (CRP), a marker in the blood of inflammation.

For years doctors have used a blood test for CRP as a way to confirm the diagnosis of inflammatory diseases such as rheumatoid arthritis. More recently, we've come to realize that even moderate elevations of CRP are associated with a high risk of developing heart disease or having a stroke.

Of all the factors that can raise your CRP level, obesity seems to lead the pack. High CRP levels are often found in obese people, suggesting that their excess weight causes a chronic, low-grade inflammation.

Unfortunately, high CRP levels are also found in people who are normal weight and appear outwardly healthy. A major study published in 1997 showed that men with the highest CRP levels had triple the risk of a future heart attack and double the risk of a stroke compared to men with the lowest CRP levels.[17]

High CRP levels are an even greater risk for women. The women most likely to have dangerously high CRP levels are menopausal women using standard hormone replacement therapy.[18] Older women in general have higher CRP concentrations than men the same age. A 1998 study of female health professionals showed that, as with men, the higher the C-reactive protein level, the greater the risk of cardiovascular events. The risk level for women was much higher, however. Women with the highest levels of CRP had 7.3 times the risk of a heart attack or stroke than those with normal CRP levels.[19]

If there is good news about CRP, it is that it predicts heart trouble very early on. Among men (we don't know about women yet), elevated levels of C-reactive protein were found to predict the risk of a first heart attack as many as six to eight years into the future. That gives you plenty of time to lose weight, get off hormone replacement therapy (if you're a woman), and institute the diet and heart-protective vitanutrient program discussed in this book.

How to Lower Your CRP Levels, Naturally

At this point, the only drug therapy that has been shown to reduce CRP levels is a daily regimen of low-dose aspirin (81 mg). The research shows that this works best for the people with the highest CRP levels.[20]

I don't like to prescribe aspirin or any of the other common nonsteroidal anti-inflammatory drugs such as ibuprofen, since the long-term side effects can be serious. Instead, I prefer to have my patients take some of the impressive array of vitanutrients that suppress inflammation, such as fish oil and GLA (see Chapter 14 for more on these). The vitanutrient most likely to lower blood markers for inflammation is MSM (methyl sulfonyl methane), a naturally occurring sulfur compound found in small amounts in a variety of fruits, vegetables, and grains. The amounts needed to treat inflammation are fairly large— some 10 grams a day or more—but MSM is extremely safe and very few if any side effects would be expected at that dose or even more.

Stealth Pathogens

Many researchers and physicians, and I am one of them, are beginning to conclude that inflammation is fundamental to the genesis of atherosclerosis. C-reactive protein is only a marker of the existence of inflammation in the blood vessels. But where there is inflammation, there is almost always also infection. Once researchers made the C-reactive protein connection, they reasoned that perhaps these patients had some sort of infection. Their thinking was borne out when many of the patients did indeed improve with antibiotic therapy.[21]

Since that initial observation, researchers have been vigorously seeking the possible infectious agent or agents. The mounting evidence from the research has narrowed the search to a handful of likely suspects. The leading culprits now seem to be two different bacteria: *Chlamydia pneumoniae* and mycoplasma. The chlamydia bacteria is related to the one that is sexually transmitted. There's also some very strong evidence that the herpes virus family, particularly a member called cyto-megalovirus (CMV), is often to blame for some cases of heart disease.

Researchers call these various microorganisms "stealth" bacteria or viruses because they are both very common and very hard to detect. They infect us without producing the usual responses to infection, such as fever or raised white blood cell count. The only way you might know you've been infected is that you now carry antibodies to one or more of the organisms in your blood. It's quite likely that at least 50 percent of the population is infected by *C. pneumoniae* at some point in their lives.[22] Cytomegalovirus is perhaps even more common. By age thirty-five, about half the population has been exposed to the virus; by age sixty, about 60 to 70 percent has been infected.[23] For many people, infection means nothing; but for some, the insidious harm these microorganisms can do may be discovered only years later.

A growing body of precedent-shattering research suggests that stealth pathogens are the underlying cause not just of some cases of heart disease but also of chronic illness such as multiple sclerosis, rheumatoid arthritis, fibromyalgia, Alzheimer's, and chronic fatigue syndrome. This research will, I believe, reveal so much about the nature of chronic illness and how it can be treated and avoided that it will be an important key to extending our life spans.

Chlamydia and Heart Disease

The connection among chlamydia, chronic heart disease, and heart attacks was first shown in 1988, but the evidence for chlamydia as a factor in the causation of heart disease is strong and growing stronger all the time. This is very significant news, because it helps us understand some baffling cases of heart disease that seem to have no cause and don't always respond well to treatment.

The Dangers of CMV

Just as we now know that the chlamydia bacterium is found inside atherosclerotic plaque, we also now know that another stealth pathogen, cytomegalovirus, is sometimes found.[24] It's entirely possible that this stealth virus causes some cases of clogged coronary arteries by infecting the arterial wall.[25]

Mycoplasma: The Stealthiest Pathogen

The class of bacteria known as mycoplasma are the stealthiest of all the stealth pathogens, for their cell walls are diminished or missing altogether. Cell-wall deficient (CWD) bacteria (to give stealth bacteria their more scientific name) enter right into your cells, where they can hide from the immune cells that circulate in your blood—and from most standard antibiotics. The nature of CWD bacteria also makes them very difficult to detect. The standard measure of infection—a raised white blood cell count—doesn't occur when you're infected with mycoplasma.

So far, we must home in on a diagnosis of mycoplasma through indirect techniques. When all the usual complementary treatments for illnesses such as chronic fatigue syndrome, multiple sclerosis, atherosclerosis, heart arrhythmias, and brain disorders fail, we must then ask if mycoplasma is the true root of the problem. In the case of heart disease, this is particularly so when the patient has no other risk factors—as is the case in a substantial percentage of all first heart attacks and many cases of heart rhythm problems and heart failure.

Treating Stealth Infections

From the perspective of a complementary practitioner, stealth pathogens present a bit of a dilemma. I am always very reluctant to prescribe antibiotics for my patients because of their serious side effects, yet one or more courses of powerful antibiotics such as doxycycline, ciprofloxacin, or azithromycin are often required to knock out the infection. That could mean months of taking drugs. While that may well heal the patient, in the larger sense it is a real quandary. We certainly don't want to risk creating a drug-resistant "superbug" or causing a yeast overgrowth in the digestive tract of the patient (see Chapter 16 for more on avoiding and treating yeast infections).

Our understanding of stealth bacteria and the best ways to treat them is still in the early stages. Part of the treatment at present includes antibiotics for patients with confirmed stealth infections. To minimize the side effects and support the patient's natural immunity, I also prescribe a number of additional vitanutrients (see Chapter 15 for more on ways to enhance your immune system).

Have I enlightened you a bit about your blood lipids? Have I gotten you outraged about homocysteine? Have I frightened you about stealth bacteria? I certainly hope so, because now you're ready to learn one of the most important lessons there is about your health. In the next chapter, I'll teach you how all these factors come together to cause heart disease—and how you can reverse the process.

4

Diabetic Heart Disease—Avoid It and Add Twelve Years

U p to this point, I've stressed four main ideas:

- Whatever causes today's heart disease epidemic was not there eighty or more years ago. Heart attacks are a modern phenomenon that occurs in Western cultures.
- Cleave's Rule of Twenty Years warns that whenever refined carbohydrates become a major addition to a culture, two diseases begin to emerge twenty years later: diabetes and coronary heart disease.
- The ratio of blood lipid levels most likely to result in a heart attack is the combination of high triglycerides and low HDL cholesterol.
- By restricting carbohydrates, my heart patients almost always report improvement in symptoms and are able to reduce or stop medications for heart disease, high blood pressure, and/or diabetes.

What do all these important facts have in common? What do they tell you about reversing heart disease?

I'll take my time explaining, but the short answer is that all these facts point to the idea that humans are generally unable to handle a lot of refined carbohydrates. When we eat a lot of desserts, bread, pasta, rice, and other highly processed starches and sugars, our ability to utilize insulin becomes impaired—we become insulin resistant and glucose intolerant. We put out excessive amounts of insulin, which in turn creates diabetes, hypertension, and atherosclerosis, the garden variety form of heart disease.

Remember the results of Cleave's research? He linked both diabetes and heart disease to the consumption of refined carbohydrates in a typical westernized diet. To summarize his work, we can say that anyone who is genetically prone to diabetes and coronary heart disease and who also eats a high-carbohydrate diet is almost certain to make that genetic tendency become manifest.

Now here's where Cleave's genius applies most. In the year 1900, a time before heart disease had become a leading cause of death, Americans consumed more carbohydrates than now, but only a relatively small part of them could be classified as refined. Back then, grains were not milled into nutritional nothingness. Even though people ate a lot of sugar then, it was often in the form of unrefined molasses, a rich source of iron and B vitamins. Most important, the fats they ate were chiefly butter and lard; trans fats hadn't been invented yet.

It's time now to learn why heart disease and diabetes are so inextricably linked; why what ultimately links them is diet, specifically a diet high in carbohydrates; and why the refining of carbohydrates is in reality the greatest *unacknowledged* cause of death in world history.

Heart Disease and Diabetes: The Link

Type II diabetes, also known as adult-onset or noninsulin diabetes, affects 95 percent of the sixteen million diabetics in

America. An additional sixty million Americans who are very likely prediabetic are afflicted, whether they know it or not, with some form of insulin disorder. These disorders progress in stages from insulin resistance to a diagnosis of full-blown diabetes. Each stage has its own findings, and even though you may not notice new symptoms, each opens a door to the range of degenerative diseases we associate with aging. So a discussion of the stages of this disease, technical though it may be, will help you understand the connections among carbohydrates, disease, and aging.

Stage 1: Insulin Resistance

In stage 1, insulin, a hormone made in your pancreas, can no longer perform its major roles in the body to a full extent. This situation is referred to as insulin resistance. Insulin's major role is to convert excess sugar (glucose) into a storage form of energy (glycogen). Glycogen is used as a fuel for later times (between meals), but excess glycogen can be converted into stored fat (triglyceride).

Insulin resistance is hard to diagnose in normal medical practice because it involves the simultaneous measurement of glucose from an artery and a vein of the same leg. Instead, we diagnose it by inference—weight gain or the finding of the second stage of diabetes.

Stage 2: Hyperinsulinism

The big breakthrough in understanding diabetes was the technology for doing serum insulin levels. Much to everyone's surprise, it was quickly discovered that type II diabetics were the polar opposite of type I insulin-dependent diabetics. Type IIs put out *too much* insulin—they have hyperinsulinism. Type I diabetics, because they have a damaged pancreas, don't put out any insulin.

Here we see the twentieth century's crosscurrents at work again. The scientific community clearly demonstrated that the two illnesses sharing the name "diabetes" were completely different illnesses, type I coming from insulin *lack* and type II deriving from insulin *resistance*. In my experience the American Diabetes Association erroneously insists that they are variants of the same disease and usually treats type II patients with insulin or insulin-releasing drugs.

Shortly after the discovery that insulin levels could be measured, it was established that excessive insulin could itself lead to heart disease and other illnesses. Dr Gerald Reaven of Stanford University summarized the impact of hyperinsulinism, to which he gave the name Syndrome X. The five major features of Syndrome X include abdominal obesity (our nation's single most prevalent abnormality, as I'm sure you've noticed), hypertension, a variety of blood sugar abnormalities, and two heart risk factors, high triglycerides and low HDL cholesterol.

Now, if you are the kind of reader who likes to form conclusions *while* you are reading, you may well have reacted to something I just wrote. Feel free to exclaim: "The link between diabetes and heart disease begins with its second stage! Diabetes causes heart disease before it is recognized as diabetes!" Congratulations—you've caught on.

Stage 3: Blood Sugar Abnormalities

Diagnosing the very common stage 3 requires a glucose tolerance test (GTT), a test of such import that I have ordered it on more than forty thousand Atkins Center patients. The GTT shows when the insulin disorder is beginning to affect the blood sugar's response to the oral intake of glucose. Sometimes, the abnormality appears at the beginning of the test when the blood glucose rises to a point higher than that of a normal person's (generally considered to be 160 mg/dL). More often, it appears on the downslope, when, presumably affected by the increased quantity or effectiveness of the insulin hyperactivity, the glucose level drops at a rate exceeding 50 points in a single hour, or 100 points in total.

Interpreting the GTT is occasionally quite subjective, but most of the time it's perfectly obvious when the criteria of abnormality are exceeded in a major way. I always administer the GTT in conjunction with a symptom questionnaire, because the symptoms of blood sugar instability as noticed by the patient are every bit as important in establishing a diagnosis as is the GTT.

You should all be aware of some of the major symptoms best explained by unstable blood sugar response. They are hour-by-hour changes in energy level, mood, brain function, and irritability brought on by being somewhat hungry and relieved by food or caffeine. Carbohydrate cravings, prominent hunger, and excessive tiredness are also commonly noted.

If your dietary habits include lots of refined carbohydrates, fruit juice, caffeine, sweets, or alcohol, the *suspicion* that you may be in the third stage (and the last prediabetic stage) may serve you just as well as the *certainty* that you do. If the suspicion leads you to change your errant ways, it will serve the desired purpose—preventing you from progressing to the next stage.

Remember this: Stage 3 is quite common. I see bona fide abnormalities in GTTs in my patients about four times more often than I see diabetes. That would suggest that there are four times more prediabetics than diabetics. Since about 8 to 9 percent of the adult American population is thought to have diabetes, this would mean that one-third of the American population has one of the stages of prediabetes. Once you know you have the problem and make the necessary dietary changes and take the appropriate vitanutrients, you are very unlikely to progress to stage 4.

Stage 4: Recognizable Type II Diabetes

There is very little difference between the typical form of type II diabetes and stage 3. No new symptoms develop, there is rarely a change in the overweight problem that plagues more than 80 percent of these people, and there is rarely a worsening of heart symptoms. The insulin resistance and hyperinsulinism that defined stages 1 through 3 are still there. It's simply that now the blood sugars are generally elevated throughout the day.

That means that type II diabetes responds to the same low-carbohydrate diet and vitanutrients that bring the prediabetic stages under control. What is the countercurrent that denies these science-based facts? Your diabetologist is almost certain to recommend continuance of your high-carbohydrate food consumption and prescribe drugs—usually including those which increase your insulin levels and may well increase your likelihood of a fatal heart attack.

Not all stage 4 diabetics continue to put out excessive insulin throughout their illness. They do, however, continue to have blood sugar elevations for the reason common to all five stages of type II: They are insulin resistant. It is not until this late stage of diabetes that insulin output begins to be inadequate—and insulin failure leads to stage 5.

Stage 5: Diabetes, Type II, with Low Insulin

Diabetologists who confuse type I with type II diabetes are justified in their error only when this stage is reached. By this point in a type II diabetic's life, his or her insulin output has finally become subnormal.

At the Atkins Center, we routinely test our type II diabetics by drawing insulin levels before and after a high-carbohydrate test meal. If there is any elevation of insulin after the breakfast, it can come only from a functioning pancreas. In our diabetic patients, only 10 percent put out insulin levels inadequate to be managed without insulin supplement.

The countercurrent? Some 44 percent of type II diabetics who consult diabetes specialists are prescribed insulin. The Atkins Center experience implies that the majority of them are given insulin unnecessarily.

At this point you might rightly raise this question: "What could be so wrong with prescribing insulin to a diabetic?" The answer has been scientifically demonstrated. If excessive insulin is harmful to an early-stage diabetic, it has been demonstrated to be equally harmful to a late-stage one.

I have never described diabetes in such detail, and I apologize if my discussion appears technical. But the information, as you will soon see, will prove important, because avoiding diabetes-related illness is likely to be the most important key to avoiding aging.

5

Insulin: The Key to Aging

So far, you've learned that:

- Most of today's premature aging comes from heart-damaging atherosclerosis.
- No human civilization ever consumed a preponderance of carbohydrates in the form of refined products with most of their original vitanutrient content discarded until the twentieth-century westernized diet became prevalent.
- There is now a worldwide epidemic of diabetes.
- There are three prediabetic stages a type II diabetic goes through prior to becoming diabetic. All of these stages are associated with excessive insulin outpouring when carbohydrates are consumed.
- People with prediabetes, or hyperinsulinism, outnumber known diabetics considerably, perhaps by four to one.
- The most predictive risk factors for atherosclerosis (high triglycerides and low HDL cholesterol) are caused primarily by hyperinsulinism.

- All of these observations have been confirmed by numerous studies by reputable scientists. Most of them have not come to the attention of the general public and certainly are not heeded by government officials or the leaders of the medical establishment.

I wonder how many of you are beginning to conclude that I will be the first physician/author to tell you the hard truth: Excessive insulin, prediabetes, and refined carbohydrates have an awfully strong connection with shortening human life spans.

Well, you're right about where my logic will take us, but I cannot claim to be the first to espouse the theory. That honor belongs to a world-famous Russian scientist, Dr. Vladimir Dilman, of St Petersburg. In a long series of books and scientific papers, Professor Dilman presented a comprehensive theory that the symptoms of aging are caused mainly by hyperinsulinism. I prefer not to go into great detail about all of Professor Dilman's theories, simply because he was such a pioneer and his work was done thirty to forty years ago. It forms the intellectual scaffolding for the vast amount of scientific research that has come since then, and I would rather present the updated results of his contributions. I will tell a little story about the man who so influenced my thinking about how to defy age.

Dr. Dilman decided to close out his career in New York City. When he arrived, he called me to introduce himself. He told me that as far as he was concerned, I was the only American doctor who seemed to be on the right track. He told me he would like to work with me in doing further research on longevity. I was more than flattered but had to inform him that the Atkins Center is not set up as a research facility—our function is strictly to help our patients get and stay well. We stayed in touch nonetheless until his untimely death just a few years before this book was written. Much of what he taught me is still quite relevant in the fight against aging, and it is my pleasure and privilege to pass it on to you.

An example of the very revealing research on aging that is going on as I write this book is the ongoing New England Centenarian Study (NECS). Researchers from Harvard University have been studying centenarian volunteers in the New England area for a number of years now, and they've come up with some very interesting results. One statistic from the study helps prove Dilman's point and mine. Of the 169 participants in the study—all of them people who have reached the age of at least one hundred in fairly good health—only *six* have diabetes. That works out to only 3 percent of the total participants.[1] These people are living examples of how important maintaining good blood sugar control is to defying aging. In this chapter I'll explain to you exactly why that's so and exactly what you have to do to control your own blood sugar.

How Sweet Goes Sour

Let's start by defining some terms. We'll begin with glucose. This is the type of sugar your body uses as the main fuel for its operations. Where does the fuel come from? Mostly from the food you eat. Your body converts the carbohydrates in that food—which either already are sugars (the simple carbohydrates) or are quickly converted to glucose (the complex carbohydrates, or starches)—into sugars. From the fats in the food that you eat, your body absorbs glycerol and fatty acids. Your body also absorbs the proteins in your diet by breaking them down into their fundamental building blocks, amino acids.

To explain what happens once glucose enters your bloodstream, I now must define the term we've been so focused on:

insulin. You've undoubtedly heard of insulin, particularly in connection with diabetes. It's the hormone your pancreas makes to control the use, distribution, and storage of energy in your body by processing blood sugar.

Insulin fuels your body by carrying glucose from your blood to your cells, where it is then carried to the mitochondria, tiny structures within the cells that act as little power plants to burn the glucose.

When you eat foods containing carbohydrates, glucose enters your bloodstream. In response to the rise in your blood sugar from eating, the portion of your pancreas known as the islets of Langerhans pours out insulin to tell all that sugar where to go. The insulin carries some of the sugar to your cells to be burned as fuel. Some of the sugar that's not needed immediately is converted to glycogen, a starch that's stored in your muscles and liver. Glycogen is your body's spare gas tank, able to provide quick energy when it's needed. The glycogen storage areas fill up pretty quickly, though. We have only a two-day, two-thousand-calorie glycogen supply. The sugar that's left in your blood at that point gets converted by insulin into tiny fat particles called triglycerides, which are what your body fat is made from and which are about as predictive a risk factor for heart disease as you can find.

So far, so good. Your body uses insulin to keep your blood sugar within a fairly narrow range, generally between 65 and 100 mg per 100 cc of blood. That's the level your body works best at, and it's the level that millions of years of evolution have designed your body to maintain.

Evolution is a very slow process, however. Your body is perfectly adapted to eat the foods that were the mainstays of existence for the vast length of human history: fats and proteins from animal foods and unrefined carbohydrates from plant foods. Fats have virtually no effect and proteins have very little effect on your blood sugar and insulin levels. Unrefined carbohydrates from fruits, vegetables, and whole grains are relatively low in carbohydrates and release their sugar slowly into your blood.*

By contrast, the typical human today eats very few unrefined carbohydrates. Instead, we eat huge amounts of refined carbohydrates, mostly in the form of sugar (especially table sugar and high-fructose corn syrup), skim milk, fruit juice, dried fruit, and refined starches (white flour in bread, baked goods, pasta, and the like). To this is added other starchy foods such as baked potatoes and white rice. This is a diet that your body was never meant to cope with. It plays havoc with your blood sugar and your insulin.

Eating the typical high-carbohydrate American diet means that your body is constantly producing large amounts of insulin to cope with all that glucose. If, like most people, you eat that diet in large portions, you're going to have a lot of leftover glucose in your blood, which your insulin will promptly convert to fat. Now the vicious cycle really sets in, because the fatter you get, the less responsive to insulin your cells become. Eating carbohydrates triggers your body to release insulin, but your cells don't want to let it in. That phenomenon is called insulin resistance. In an effort to maintain its normal equilibrium, your body then produces even more insulin to overcome the resistance.

Because the insulin can't carry much glucose to your cells to be burned as fuel, the glucose remains in your blood. Insulin converts some of the excess sugar to fat instead. You get fatter, and you also feel tired all the time, partly because your cells aren't getting the fuel they need, and partly because the excess

*How slowly varies, depending on the food. The effect of individual foods on your sugar and insulin levels is quantified by a system called the glycemic index. See the appendix for the glycemic index values of a variety of foods.

insulin drives your blood sugar levels below the optimal range. Your body can't convert all that excess sugar into fat fast enough to keep it from circulating in your blood. As I'll explain later on in this chapter, excess sugar in the blood is very damaging. Your heart, blood vessels, kidneys, eyes, and nerves are particularly vulnerable.

As you slide farther down the slippery slope of insulin resistance, you're putting out insulin all the time, yet it's not doing you much good. In fact, it's doing serious damage to your body. You've developed hyperinsulinism: Your insulin output is always too high even as your body is resistant to its effects. That equates to the second stage of type II diabetes, as I described in Chapter 4. The next step from there will be abnormalities on a glucose tolerance test (stage 3) and a very probable progression to type II diabetes (stage 4).

If you're not overweight, you're probably thinking, "Well, I'm safe. No blood sugar worries for me." I'm sorry to tell you that you're not safe at all. The mere fact of growing older means your cells are becoming at least somewhat resistant to glucose. About 25 percent of all apparently healthy, normal-weight adults are affected by insulin resistance. Among people who smoke and/or have a sedentary lifestyle, the percentage is even higher. The next step up, impaired glucose tolerance, is said to affect 11 percent of the healthy adult population, but I believe the number is actually considerably more. In my experience, which includes reviewing more than forty-five thousand glucose tolerance tests, abnormal glucose responses outnumber diabetes by four to one. This implies that nearly half of all adults, by the time they reach the age of fifty, will demonstrate at least some instability in their blood sugar and at least some insulin resistance. Of course, if you're considerably overweight, your chances of having insulin resistance, hyperinsulinism, and eventual diabetes are approaching near certainty.

The Aging Express Lane

It comes down to this: Hyperinsulinism accelerates aging. Even small elevations in glucose and insulin levels affect your health as you age and are closely related to the chronic disorders of aging, including heart disease, cancer, and diabetes.[2]

It's not just an issue of normal versus abnormal—there are many gradations of glucose and insulin levels. For instance, if your fasting glucose is in the upper range of normal, you have a substantially higher risk of death from heart disease than someone at the lower end of normal. In fact, if you're a middle-aged man with a fasting blood glucose level between 85 and 109 mg/dL, your heart risk is 40 percent higher than average. You also have a greater chance of several other unfavorable cardiovascular risk factors, including high blood pressure and high LDL cholesterol and triglycerides.[3] If you have gone beyond simply being at the high end to having impaired glucose tolerance, meaning that your fasting blood glucose level is above 110 mg/dL but not yet at the diabetic level of above 125, you're at even greater risk for cardiovascular disease.[4] I'm sure future studies will confirm that insulin gradations within the normal range are just as predictive of these problems as is glucose. For most people, glucose and insulin vary together.

Now that I've explained some of the terms I use, we should scrutinize the ways glucose intolerance and hyperinsulinism affect how you age.

How Sugar Makes Us AGE

I told you that elevated blood sugar levels are bad for you. I told you that diabetics don't live as long as other people and that very few centenarians are diabetics—but I didn't tell you why. The "because" that answers this particular "why" is worth your attention. It's because of the adverse effect that blood sugar elevations have on our body's organs. The process whereby sugar does that is called glycosylation. Once you know how glycosylation can hurt you, you may never enjoy another dessert again. The process has been well researched, but it's not well known to the general public, so let me try to explain it to you.

Sugar is sticky, as you discover every time you spill some and have to wipe it up. When you have extra sugar floating around in your bloodstream, those sticky glucose molecules attach themselves to proteins. The sugar attachment to protein is the process I referred to as glycosylation (also called glycation). When glucose attaches to protein in places where it doesn't belong, it sets in motion a slow chain of chemical reactions that ends with the proteins binding together, or cross-linking, and forming a new chemical structure. The brilliant biochemist Anthony Cerami, who discovered the glycosylation process in living tissue, gave these new structures a very apt name: Advanced Glycosylation End-products, or AGEs.

Why are AGEs so dangerous? Because what's happening to your tissues from exposure to excess glucose is exactly what happens to meat when you brown it. You're slowly cooking yourself from the inside. Glycosylation alters the very structure of proteins and keeps them from doing what they're supposed to. Collagen is one of the first proteins to be affected. Collagen is the tough but flexible connective tissue that holds your skeleton together, attaches your muscles to your bones, and is the foundation of all your blood vessels, skin, lungs, and cartilage. When collagen becomes glycosylated, AGEs form. The cross-linking destroys collagen's flexibility, which means that your blood vessels, lungs, and joints all stiffen and your skin sags. AGEs also cloud the proteins in the lens of your eye, causing cataracts.

Other proteins are also affected by AGEs. Glucose easily combines with the protein hemoglobin in your blood—in fact, that's the basis of a valuable blood test for diabetes, called glycosylated hemoglobin (GHb). GHb measures the average blood sugar you have been running for several consecutive months. It gives an indication of how much AGEing you have done during that time.

AGEs affect production of the more than fifty thousand different proteins your body makes to regulate its functions. Among them are the antioxidant enzymes that protect you against free radicals (dangerous unpaired electrons, which I discuss at length in Chapter 6). When glucose attaches to these enzymes, they are inactivated. Many other proteins are part of complex chemical cascades that send messages around your body, turn genes on and off, repair damage, and control the growth and replication of cells. When these controlling proteins are damaged by AGEs, the chemical messages are garbled or don't get through at all. The proper functioning of a cell is disrupted, which in turn causes further disruption down the line. If the disruption causes a gene to switch on or off inappropriately, or tells a cell to replicate when it shouldn't, the process that leads to cancer and other problems is initiated. It's possible that AGEs can even bind directly to the DNA in a cell's nucleus. Although the process would happen very slowly, over the long run it would cause serious damage in cells that don't reproduce, like the ones in your heart and brain.

Sticky AGEs tend to form clumps of cross-linked proteins, clumps that are very similar to the tangles and plaques that are found in the brains of Alzheimer's patients. Indeed, AGEs have been found in these plaques at about three times the level of normal brains, suggesting that they are responsible, at least in part, for the progression of this dreadful disease.[5]

When glucose attaches to peptides, tiny protein molecules,

the resulting AGEs end up circulating in your blood. This can have a very bad effect on your blood lipids, because the AGE-modified peptides can then attach to molecules of LDL cholesterol. Recent research suggests that your body can no longer recognize this new substance as being LDL. Instead of being removed from your blood as part of the normal clearance process, the LDL stays in circulation. The research explains in part why diabetics have such dangerously high levels of LDL cholesterol—all the extra sugar in their blood leads to high levels of circulating AGEs.[6]

Your body does have some natural defenses against AGEs. At least one type of scavenger cell of your immune system engulfs and destroys AGEs, but the process doesn't seem to be very efficient, and it slows down with age. Your antioxidant enzymes may also play a part in keeping AGEs to a minimum. Interestingly, AGEs may explain the beneficial effect on the heart of having a daily glass of wine or a cocktail. The alcohol seems to block the formation of some AGEs at an intermediate stage in the process, keeping them from building up inside your arteries and damaging your LDL cholesterol.[7]

Free Radicals: Hastening the Aging Process

In the next chapter, I'll be pointing out to you that the free radical theory of aging is perhaps the most widely accepted explanation for the aging process. Anything that causes you to produce an excess of free radicals will cause you to age more rapidly; similarly, anything that reduces your level of antioxidants to fight off those free radicals will also cause faster aging.

Before I establish the major role free radicals play in the aging process, I must point out that both insulin resistance and impaired glucose tolerance will increase free radicals and weaken your antioxidant defense. There is abundant evidence that excess insulin and excess sugar in the blood cause you to produce large numbers of free radicals—more than your body can cope with. Indeed, the overabundance of free radicals is one of the primary reasons for the accelerated aging often seen in diabetics. Even slight elevations in your blood sugar are enough to produce excess free radicals. And because vitamin C is carried into your cells along with insulin, one consequence of even slight insulin resistance is that you'll have less of this powerful antioxidant in your cells. AGEs also reduce your level of antioxidant enzymes by inactivating them and damaging the mechanism that creates them.

Hyperinsulinism and Hypertension

Here's another way that insulin resistance and glucose intolerance conspire to age you: They raise your blood pressure. It's well known that one of the most serious consequences of diabetes is sharply raised blood pressure and thus a far greater risk of heart disease, stroke, and kidney disease. There's no doubt that an elevated insulin response is one of the major causes of hypertension. Indeed, Stanford's Dr. Gerald Reaven, a leading researcher in this area, feels that a plethora of scientific studies establish that 60 percent of hypertension cases can be attributed to hyperinsulinism. You certainly don't have to be diabetic to get blood pressure elevations; the insulin disorders that appear long before diabetes will do the trick.[8]

A conventional doctor will probably tell you that your blood pressure is going up simply because you're getting older. Indeed, elevated blood pressure among older adults is so common that it's called age-related hypertension. When it happens to you, you've reached the stage in life that the drug companies love. They feel they can get you to become a lifelong customer for medications that lower blood pressure, including diuretics and beta-blockers. But, when it comes to these drugs, even prescription ones, the answer still is, "Just say no." I've treated more than ten thousand patients who were taking blood pressure medications. Nutritional changes—a new diet and vita-nutrients—allowed them to get off their medications. We consistently bring high blood pressure right back down to normal by reducing the carbohydrates in your diet (which returns your blood glucose and insulin to better levels) and adding vita-nutrients such as taurine, magnesium, potassium, coenzyme Q_{10}, hawthorn, and garlic. Of course, if you're overweight, shedding those excess pounds (the automatic consequence of cutting carbohydrates) will also help return your blood pressure to normal.

DHEA Disturbances

In Chapter 12, I will present DHEA (dehydroepiandrosterone) as a critically important hormone for defying the aging process. For the present, I would merely like to point out that a rising insulin level causes your DHEA to drop.

Here too, the effects are seen long before diabetes develops. If you're at the high end of normal, lowering your insulin level will still increase your DHEA level.[9]

If your DHEA levels are high, you're much less likely to develop diabetes to begin with. That's because DHEA improves insulin resistance, even in people who already have diabetes.[10] Interestingly, chromium picolinate, a supplement we often use at the Atkins Center to improve the insulin resistance of diabetic patients, also seems to increase your production of DHEA by lowering your blood levels of insulin.[11]

One of the best ways to maintain a high **DHEA** level is to keep your insulin level low, because insulin, more than anything else, will suppress your natural **DHEA** production.

The Consequences of Insulin Resistance

By now you should be acutely aware of what happens when you develop insulin resistance. All the degenerative diseases common to aging are given an opportunity to worsen your health. Atherosclerosis, hypertension, diabetes, obesity, cancer, impaired immunity—all these health problems are said to be aging changes, an inevitable part of growing older.

Are they? Certainly not. In almost all cases the multiple adverse changes of age I just listed are really the accumulated consequences of high blood sugar and high insulin. They are far from inevitable—indeed, they can be prevented and even reversed. How? By keeping your blood sugar and insulin levels at the lower end of normal through a diet that is low in carbohydrates and high in antioxidants and vitanutrients.

When you get to Part III of this book, you will learn exactly how this can be done. For now, let's look at the other prominent theories about the causes of aging. Any valid cause will have to be defied, so let's see what they are.

6

Free Radicals: The Heart of the Matter

There are a lot of issues that my colleagues in antiaging medicine disagree on, but there's one that has near unanimous agreement: *Damage from free radicals is at the heart of aging.* Please take a moment to reread that sentence, then memorize it.

Avoiding, minimizing, and counteracting the damaging effects of free radicals must be the fundamental principle of any age-defying program. Everything and anything you do to reduce the damage from free radicals will do that much more to give you the best chance possible of living to your full life span with a minimum of disability.

The free radical theory of aging is so central to my age-defying diet that I'm using this chapter to explain it and begin the discussion of how you can minimize the damage. In this chapter I'll explain the basic concepts behind the free radical theory of aging and how damage from free radicals accumulates and causes aging. Without understanding this basic concept, you won't be able to fully grasp the concepts I'll be discussing in the rest of this book. I'll discuss the agents for controlling free radicals through vitanutrients and the very foods you eat in Chapters 19 through 22.

The Free Radical Theory of Aging

Today we're on the threshold of a revolution in medicine, led by the great researcher Dr. Denham Harman. His revolutionary concept, first proposed in 1954 and ignored by most of the scientific establishment for some twenty years, is the Free Radical Theory of Aging (FRTA).[1] Essentially, Harman's theory states that free radical reactions—a normal and unavoidable aspect of your metabolism—are the cause of the slow deterioration of your body over time. In other words, you age because free radicals damage your cells. Free radicals are especially likely to damage your mitochondria, the tiny energy-producing structures within your cells. The more damage to your mitochondria, the faster you age and the more likely you are to develop an age-related disease such as high blood pressure or cancer.[2]

Harman's free radical theory, once it is finally accepted by the medical profession, will eventually lead to the slowing or elimination of age-related illnesses, which in turn may well lead to huge increases in life span. Living in good health to the age of one hundred and beyond will become not just possible but common. Dr. Harman, who is now over eighty and is a professor emeritus of medicine at the University of Nebraska, is the recipient of many honors, which I feel are just the beginning of the universal acclamation he deserves.

Free Radicals and Your Health

I wouldn't be surprised if you've been hearing a lot about free radicals from sources other than me—I'm not the only doctor who gets on the radio and writes books. Like most well-informed people interested in health, you probably have at least a rough idea of what a free radical is, but the concept is so important that I want to go into it in some detail here. I'll save the specific details of how your diet and supplements affect free radicals for later chapters.

Understanding Free Radicals

Let's start by defining a free radical. You'll remember from high school chemistry class that an atom consists of a nucleus surrounded by pairs of negatively charged electrons orbiting around it. If one of the electrons in a pair is stripped away, the atom (or the molecule of which the atom is part) becomes unstable. It becomes highly reactive as it seeks to restore its energy balance by grabbing on to another electron—any electron from anywhere. A highly reactive, out-of-balance atom or molecule with one or more unpaired electrons is known as a free radical.

Almost all living things, including plants, need oxygen to live. Every single cell in your body uses oxygen to create energy—without oxygen, the cell will die. In your cells, energy is produced by tiny structures called mitochondria. The process is quite complex, but what's important here is that free radicals are a necessary part of it. Most of the free radicals are contained within the process and neutralized instantly, but even so, quite a few escape. A good analogy is the way your car burns gasoline and oxygen in the pistons to produce the energy that drives it—but also produces waste products such as water vapor and carbon monoxide. When your body burns oxygen to create energy, the waste products are water and oxygen-based free radicals, also known as reactive oxygen species.

When a free radical escapes, it goes scurrying around in

your body's cells looking for another electron. It might grab the electron from the cell membrane, or perhaps from some other structure in the cell, such as the DNA contained in the nucleus. You might not think the loss of a single electron could do much damage, especially when you know that your body has about sixty trillion cells in it. But every moment of every day, every one of those cells is producing millions of free radicals, and when a free radical grabs an electron from a nearby molecule, the process doesn't stop there. Not only is the molecule damaged, but another free radical has now been created. The process sets off a cascade of more free radicals that damage more healthy molecules. To use another automotive analogy, one free radical can be like the nail in the road that punctures your tire. You swerve and crash into another car, which then crashes into another car, and so on, until the process finally stops when no more cars come along. What's left is a pile-up of smashed vehicles. In your body, what's left are a lot of damaged cells. The cumulative damage over years causes the diseases of aging.

Some free radical types are particularly dangerous. The superoxide free radical is created when oxygen is metabolized into ATP and water in your mitochondria. Even after the superoxide radical grabs an electron, it's still dangerous. In its reduced form, the superoxide radical goes on to react with hydrogen atoms and form hydrogen peroxide. Technically, hydrogen peroxide isn't a free radical, but it can trigger the formation of lots more free radicals. If those free radicals then react with iron or copper in your body, they produce an extremely reactive and very dangerous free radical called hydroxyl.[3]

Free Radical Damage

When free radicals attack, the damage can happen to any part of a cell. If the free radical attacks the fatty acids of the cell membrane, the cell can rupture. If the free radicals attack tiny enzyme storage structures in your cells called lysosomes, the enzymes get released into the cell and destroy it—and also nearby cells. That's bad enough, but even worse is the process known as lipid peroxidation. Free radicals attack the fatty tissues throughout your body, including the tiny cholesterol droplets that float in your blood. When free radicals attack the "bad" low-density cholesterol (LDL), it gets oxidized. The result is that the cholesterol turns much stickier—so sticky that it then attaches to rough spots on the walls of your arteries. When that happens, plaque begins to form and you're on the way to clogged arteries and a heart attack or stroke.

The DNA found in the nuclei of all your cells contains your genetic code. If it gets attacked by free radicals, the DNA that controls the cell's replication can be damaged. Another possibility is that the free radical could fuse the DNA with other proteins in the cell. Cross-linking, as this is called, means the cell can't replicate at all. In either case, the result could be cancer.

Most serious of all is free radical damage to your mitochondria. Your mitochondria have their own separate DNA that codes for the production of the thirteen mitochondrial proteins you need for cellular respiration. The DNA in the nuclei of your cells is intricately coiled and carefully packaged. Mitochondrial DNA is far more vulnerable—it's just a simple, almost unprotected ring.

Some of the superoxide free radicals used in cell respiration escape in the process—and as we grow older, more and more get away. The first organic structures they encounter are the fatty membranes of the mitochondria and the mitochondrial DNA. That means the mitochondria themselves are the most likely part of the cell to be damaged. Lipid peroxidation of the membranes can slow down or even stop energy production.

It all comes down to this, courtesy of Dr. Harman: "It is likely that the life span of an individual is primarily determined by the rate of mitochondria damage, inflicted at an increasing rate with age by free radicals arising in the mitochondria in the course of normal respiration."[4] Eventually, as your mitochondria become less efficient from accumulated free radicals, a vicious cycle begins. You produce more and more superoxide radicals and have less and less defense against them. Finally, your body's various defense mechanisms are overwhelmed.

Other Sources of Free Radicals

Interestingly, your immune system harnesses the destructive power of free radicals to destroy invaders. Your white blood cells attack invading pathogens by engulfing them and then blasting them with superoxide and hydrogen peroxide. Any illness or infection creates a lot of extra free radicals, though, so the longer you're sick, the more free radicals you create and the more damage they can do.

Many prescription drugs produce huge amounts of free radicals as they break down in your body or make your liver produce a lot of extra free radicals as it tries to metabolize the drugs. Even worse, many prescription and nonprescription drugs seriously deplete your antioxidant levels, depriving you of your natural defenses.

The foods you eat have a major effect on your production of free radicals. A big culprit here is polyunsaturated fat, especially when it's in the form of partially hydrogenated vegetable oil—the deadly *trans* fat. In Chapter 14 I will explain just how dangerous trans fats are, so here I'll just remind you that consuming trans fats is guaranteed to make you produce more free radicals.

Free radicals are generated by your liver as part of the normal detoxification process that removes waste products from your body. Free radicals are also generated in your body when you're exposed to normal background radiation and ultraviolet light from sunshine. Millions of years of evolution have made your body able to squelch most—though not all—of those free radicals. What you're not very good at is dealing with all the pollutants that accompany life in the twenty-first century, including pesticides, herbicides, ozone, smog, cigarette smoke, soot, automobile exhaust, and an increasingly wide variety of industrial chemicals. Exposure to all these pollutants creates free radicals as your body tries to expel them.

It's also important to remember that exercise produces a lot of free radicals. In fact, it's not uncommon for highly conditioned athletes such as marathon runners to get sick a lot with colds and infections. These people train so hard and produce so many free radicals that they actually damage their own immune system.

Antioxidants to the Rescue

There are basically two ways you can reduce free radical damage. The first way is to prevent the formation of excess free radicals to begin with. So far, only one thing is said to lower your production of free radicals: caloric restriction. The idea is that if you eat a lot less, you burn less fuel and create fewer free radicals. The caloric restriction theory is talked and written about more than any other antiaging theory, so I'll be discussing it in the next chapter.

A more reasonable approach is to avoid situations that increase free radical production, as I've just discussed. That means avoiding pollutants and exercising moderately. Most important, it means staying healthy and thus avoiding the double whammy of generating extra free radicals not only from illness but also from the drugs you take to help the illness.

Breaking the Chains

The most practical way to prevent free radical damage is to neutralize them rapidly and thereby break the chain reaction process as quickly as possible. By quenching free radicals just as soon as they're formed, you minimize the damage they can do. The chain-breaking approach is the very core of my age-defying program.

To break the chains of free radical damage and liberate yourself to achieve your maximum life span, you must take a two-pronged approach: Consume a diet high in antioxidant foods, and take supplements of antioxidant vitanutrients.

Having said that, it's now time to explain exactly what an antioxidant is. Antioxidants are substances your body produces to protect itself against the harmful effects of free radicals. An antioxidant is a substance that quenches a free radical by donating to it the electron it seeks. The antioxidant stops the free radical in its tracks and halts the cascade of further free radical formation.

One reason humans have much longer life spans than other animals may be that we have extremely efficient antioxidant mechanisms. They're all designed to put a quick end to the free radical chain reaction. Your first line of defense is the powerful antioxidant enzymes your body makes, including superoxide dismutase (SOD), glutathione, and catalase. They're so important that we need to take a closer look at them.

Antioxidant Enzymes and Vitanutrients

Let's start with SOD. This is the enzyme that neutralizes the superoxide free radical, the free radical that's produced so abundantly in your mitochondria. SOD interrupts the free radical chain reaction by breaking the superoxide radical down into oxygen and hydrogen peroxide. That's the first step. The next step is to break up the hydrogen peroxide, because it's a free radical, too, even though it's much less damaging than the superoxide radical. To break down the hydrogen peroxide, your body uses another enzyme, called catalase, that turns the hydrogen peroxide into plain water and oxygen. The catch here is that catalase works only in the watery parts of your body—inside your cells and outside your cells, but not in the fatty cell membranes. That's where the antioxidant enzyme glutathione comes in. It captures the free radicals attacking your cell membranes—and also picks up any hydrogen peroxide your catalase misses. That's important, because hydrogen peroxide can break down into hydroxyl, the most dangerous free radical of all. Unfortunately, your body doesn't have an enzyme system for getting rid of hydroxyl. The major natural way that your body deals with it is by neutralizing it with the natural hormone melatonin. But as you'll learn in Chapter 9, your production of melatonin drops as you age. We can and do raise it with supplements, but another way to keep melatonin levels up is to prevent hydroxyl radicals from forming.

We know from research that gets more definitive all the time that vitanutrients are essential for free radical protection. Antioxidant nutrients such as vitamin E, vitamin C, and beta-carotene protect your cells from free radicals by quenching them directly or by being essential elements in making the enzymes that do. Vitamin E is particularly helpful for protecting your cell membranes. Vitamin C is a potent antioxidant—and because it's water soluble, it can go everywhere inside and outside your cells. But don't let me get ahead of myself. You'll be reading about all the antioxidant vitanutrients later.

Many compounds found naturally in plant foods are extremely valuable for quenching the free radicals that are produced when your liver removes toxins and wastes from your body. You'll read about that too, especially in Chapter 11.

Because enzymes are made of proteins, you also need amino acids, the building blocks of proteins, to make them. You can't make glutathione, for example, without N-acetyl cysteine (NAC), a form of the amino acid cysteine. You also need a good supply of trace minerals to make antioxidant enzymes. Take selenium as an example. You need it to make glutathione—not enough selenium, not enough glutathione. Likewise, you need iron to make catalase, and zinc, copper, and manganese to make SOD.

Eating all the good foods in the world won't help your antioxidant levels if you're also taking drugs that suppress them. There's a very long list of drugs that, in my opinion, can deplete the trace minerals and vitamins you need to manufacture antioxidant enzymes. I'll just mention a few here. Over-the-counter medications such as antacids and antihistamines can block your use of antioxidants and let the free radicals run wild. Prescription drugs such as broad-spectrum antibiotics can also have a very negative effect on your antioxidant levels as can the corticosteroids. If you're on a cortisone-type drug make sure you check out Chapter 13 on natural hormones for even more reasons not to be taking it—and ways to get off it.

The Next Steps

I know you'd like to learn what active steps you can take to protect yourself against free radicals, so I'll get quite specific about antioxidant vitanutrients and foods shortly. For now, just remember that you must be certain to have a good supply of the vitanutrients your body needs to produce the essential antioxidant enzymes.

Let me elaborate on this by presenting Dr. Harman's explanation for why Americans are living longer, healthier lives than ever before. He wrote in 1999: "The increases in the percentage of elderly people in the population since 1960 and the declining incidence of chronic disability among them, decreases in cancer mortality since 1991, and continuing declines in cardiovascular disease are in accord with the beneficial effects expected from the growing use of antioxidant supplements since the 1960s . . . as well as the growing publicity about the ability of fruits and vegetables to decrease disease incidence by depressing free radical reaction damage."[5]

Note carefully what Dr. Harman is saying here. The advances in longevity and health in the past few decades are due more to diet and vitanutrients than to anything the medical establishment has done. I would like next to fill you in on another major theory of aging, and then introduce you to a variety of techniques I and my colleagues use to keep people healthy, the best way I know to also keep them long-lived.

7

Caloric Restriction—and Why You Shouldn't Do It

N o discussion of antiaging theories can be complete without telling you about the most well-researched and well-documented theory of how to extend your life span: the concept of restricting our total caloric intake.

You might be a little surprised to see the idea of caloric restriction in something I write. After all, my very successful approach to weight loss is based on the idea that caloric restriction is an unacceptable activity. Here, the kind of caloric restriction I'm talking about isn't a weight-loss approach—it's a way to extend your life span. Documented or not, I still think it's a terrible idea. Indeed, when discussing this not very thrilling option, one wag opined, "You may not live to be 100, but you'll be hungry enough that it'll sure *seem* like it."

The concept of caloric restriction—a diet that's low in calories but still contains all the essential nutrients—was first proposed by Roy Walford, a researcher at UCLA. Actually, Walford describes caloric restriction as "undernutrition without malnutrition."[1] According to him, if you eat fewer calories, you'll burn less oxygen in your mitochondria, which in turn means you'll produce fewer free radicals. Walford's theory, then, would seem to tie in closely with Denham Harman's theory that accumulated free radical damage is the major cause of aging.

Of Mice and Monkeys

Caloric restriction has been shown to extend the life of lab mice and rats by nearly 50 percent.[2] In fact, caloric restriction is the *only* thing that has been proved to extend the life span of experimental animals. People aren't lab rats, of course, so it's not clear if caloric restriction would extend a human's life span.

Despite a lot of hungry rats, no one has yet shown exactly why caloric restriction extends life spans or how it works. There's no convincing proof that it works by reducing the animals' lifetime production of free radicals, although many researchers think that's the underlying reason.

Recently, though, researchers have suggested that the real benefit of caloric restriction may come simply from a reduction in body fat, which in turn decreases the amount of the various hormones and other chemical messengers body fat secretes.[3] Since many of those substances play a role in causing health problems such as insulin resistance, what all the caloric restriction experiment may be proving is something we've known for a long time: Being normal weight is healthier in general than being overweight.

I've never seen an antiaging theory so well documented with studies on lab rodents. All the studies show that caloric restriction—sometimes to levels that are less than half of the quantities the animals usually take in—extends their life spans significantly. On average, lab rats and mice that are restricted to only 60 to 70 percent of the amount control rats eat live 25 to 40 percent longer. They also appear younger and healthier for longer, with fewer tumors and higher levels of disease-fighting white blood cells.

On the other hand, calorically restricted rats have higher levels of stress hormones. If you've ever gone on the sort of low-calorie diet recommended by the medical establishment, you can understand why. The stress doesn't seem to be so severe that it hurts the rats, but nobody really knows. Maybe if the rats got somewhat more food they'd produce fewer stress hormones and do equally well.

Studies are going on right now of caloric restriction in monkeys, and the results are similar to those with rats. The calorically restricted monkeys are healthier and more youthful looking than those on the regular diet. They're also a lot hungrier. Since monkeys live on average about twenty to thirty years, it's far too soon to say if caloric restriction will actually extend their lives.

Hungry Humans

Roy Walford is experimenting on himself by restricting his caloric intake, but there's very little information on how well caloric restriction works in humans. I seriously doubt that anyone could stick to this sort of diet for very long, no matter how much longer it might help you live. It certainly isn't much of a normal life—you're a little hungry all the time, as Roy Walford himself admits in interviews.

Biologically there is very little similarity between lab rats and humans. Although humans and monkeys are closer relatives, there are still important differences. What applies to the diets of rats and monkeys in laboratory conditions just doesn't have much application to the diets of humans in the real world.

Also, it's easy to design a standard diet, calorically restricted or otherwise, for lab animals that have been bred for decades for uniformity and live in carefully controlled conditions. It's much, much harder to come up with a standard diet that's good for all humans, with our infinite variability in size, metabolism, genetic makeup, and activity level.

Let's not confuse malnutrition with deliberate undernutrition. The Walford diet contains all the nutrients you need to sustain healthy life—it just doesn't have many calories. The point is, how many of us would really want to live that way, even if it did extend our life spans? And would it? Statistical evidence from the ongoing Nurses' Health Study of more than one hundred thousand women shows that leaner isn't necessarily healthier. In fact, the difference in death rates between lean and plump women of the same height and age was negligible. Only the obese women—women 20 percent or more over their ideal weights—had a significantly higher risk of death.[4]

Dieting Without Hunger

But do you have to undereat to be at your normal weight? Of course not, as anyone who's ever read one of my other books knows. There's an easy, realistic way to get the main benefits of caloric restriction without going hungry and counting the minutes until your next meager ration. In fact, the one way to go through life eating fewer calories and *not* being constantly hungry is significantly to restrict the carbohydrates in your diet.

As I write this chapter, I keep thinking back to the crucial research paper that gave me a central insight into diet. Written in 1963 by Dr. Walter Lyons Bloom and Dr. Gordon Azar, it described the similarity between carbohydrate (not caloric) restriction and fasting.[5]

Their basic premise started with the observation that after two days of fasting, people feel very little hunger; the authors then showed that the same lack of hunger can be achieved merely by eliminating carbohydrates from the diet. Why? Because your body can store only a couple thousand calories of carbohydrate as glycogen. When that gets used up, your body automatically switches over to burning your stored fat. All the fat-mobilizing enzymes and hormones your body puts out when the switch takes place combine to cut down your appetite and reduce hunger.

To lose weight or even keep yourself at your current healthy weight, you don't need to count calories, much less restrict them. By eating intelligently based on the information in this book, you'll fill up quickly on tasty, satisfying, and nutrient-dense food. You won't feel the need to stuff yourself with carbohydrate-laden junk. If you bothered to count, you might find that you were eating somewhat fewer calories, but that doesn't matter. It's the quality of your calories, not the number of them, that makes the difference.

I've concentrated, so far, on presenting you with the rather impressive theoretical background behind the system we use at the Atkins Center to help our patients forestall the ravages of aging.

Now is the time to begin showing you how the process can be applied to you, as an individual. I stress your uniqueness, because the one-program-fits-all approach has never worked, nor can it ever work.

We'll start by learning about the many antioxidants that prevent the damage free radicals can do. Indeed, there are so many of these valuable substances that I'll spend all of Part III explaining them to you.

Part III

Age-Defying Nutrients

Antioxidants are the key to defying age. In this part I'll explain in detail how antioxidants prevent or block damage from free radicals.

■

Vitamins such as vitamin C and vitamin E are your first line of defense against free radicals.

■

Vitanutrients help your body produce its own antioxidant enzymes by providing the needed raw materials.

■

Carotenoids and bioflavonoids—antioxidants found naturally in many vegetables and fruits—are powerful weapons against aging.

8

Antioxidants Are "Vital" Nutrients

I hope my nonscientist readers will forgive me for getting technical in describing the free radical theory of aging in such detail. To me, it is inescapable that neutralizing free radical damage is pivotal to any strategy for defying aging. The technical language is consistent with my fervent wish that many copies of this book will be used to convince other doctors—your doctors—that a sophisticated knowledge of nutrition will lead to successes in turning back the clock.

You will recall that the previous chapter concluded with the idea that antioxidants, both from supplements and from foods, are the antidotes to free radicals. And now, for the same reasons my free radical discussion was technical and detailed, I'm going to spend the next four chapters telling you about antioxidants.

If this gives you the impression that I consider antioxidants to be one of the major answers to aging, I won't argue with you. But there is another reason these remarkable nutrients require so much space. Virtually every antioxidant supplement or food helps us in many ways beyond its role as an antioxidant. Thus, when I talk about these extremely valuable vitanutrients, I want you to see the many ways they can help you.

All my successful patients achieved their accomplishments with a well-thought-out program of diet and vitanutrients. I assume that my readers will require something quite similar. Please scrutinize the suggestions you'll be reading about here— most of them will apply to you.

There's no question in my mind that antioxidant vitanutrients such as vitamin C and vitamin E are crucial to your health and longevity. What I don't understand is why there's still any question in the mind of any other physician. Over the past few years, major articles about the benefits of antioxidant vitamins have appeared even in those fortresses of the medical establishment, *The New England Journal of Medicine* and *Journal of the American Medical Association*. To take just one example: A 1995 study showed, through the use of angiograms (X-ray visualizations of the heart and its blood vessels), that taking antioxidant vitamins can slow the progression of coronary artery disease by slowing plaque buildup. The vitamins work by preventing free radical damage to the LDL cholesterol in the blood.[1]

You couldn't ask for better evidence—and it was published in the *Journal of the American Medical Association*, which in my view has often been the house organ for those advocating anti-nutrition arguments in medicine.

Likewise, study after study proves that vitamin E is a significant antioxidant that fights off atherosclerosis, protects your eyesight, and prevents cancer. Yet despite the clear and convincing evidence that vitamin E has life-or-death importance to your health, your conventional doctor may not suggest taking it—even though he's likely to be taking it himself. Why might someone pledged to preserving the health of patients deprive them of such a valuable vitanutrient? It may be because, among other reasons, the American Heart Association has said so. Here's what the AHA told physicians and the public as recently as January 1999: "Although diet alone may not provide the levels of Vitamin E intake that have been associated with lowest risk in a few observational studies, the absence of efficacy and safety data from randomized trials precludes the establishment of population-wide recommendations regarding Vitamin E supplementation."

Despite the very powerful evidence in favor of antioxidant vitanutrients, and even though it's been repeatedly presented in the journals that every physician reads and relies on, your doctor might not tell you anything about how antioxidant vitanutrients can prevent free radical damage.

That's my job.

Your Prime Antioxidants

Let's start by taking a look at the major circulating antioxidant vitamins and minerals: vitamin E, vitamin C, lipoic acid, and selenium. These are the vitanutrients your body needs to mount its primary defense against free radicals, to say nothing of all the other important things they do for you.*

By themselves, each vitanutrient is a powerful free radical fighter. They're also essential elements in the antioxidant enzymes such as SOD, catalase, and glutathione that your cells make to neutralize free radicals. (I'll discuss these powerful enzymes in the next chapter. I'll get into the carotenoids, a group of related vitanutrients that includes beta-carotene, lycopene, and other valuable antioxidants, in Chapter 10.) If you don't have enough of the right vitamins and minerals to go around, you can't make enough of the enzymes—and the free radicals get the upper hand.

*For detailed information, please see *Dr. Atkins' Vita-Nutrient Solution*

By keeping your levels of these vitanutrients high, you protect yourself against the free radical damage that leads to heart disease, stroke, cancer, and memory loss and other cognitive problems. You also protect yourself against inflammatory arthritis[2] and sight-robbing cataracts and macular degeneration. And, of course, you counteract the free radical cause of aging itself.

The crucial point to remember about these antioxidants is that they work both individually and as a team. For example, whenever a molecule of vitamin E or vitamin C neutralizes a free radical, the vitamin molecule itself becomes a free radical—although one that's far less dangerous. In a complex cycle, vitamin C, vitamin E, selenium, and lipoic acid interact to regenerate the vitamins, which extends their useful life in your body and lets them get back to work.

What the antioxidant cycle shows is that no one antioxidant is a miracle cure for all your ills. To maintain good health, you need them all.

Now let's put it all together and look at how these antioxidants protect your health as you get older.

Preventing Heart Disease

There's no question that high levels of antioxidant vitamins prevent or slow heart disease. The evidence is very powerful. I'll start by looking just at the most compelling evidence for vitamin E:

• The long-running Harvard-based Physician's Health Study showed in 1993 that men who take just 100 IU of vitamin E daily have nearly half the risk of coronary artery disease as men who get less than 7 IU daily.[3]

• Likewise, the long-running Nurses' Health Study showed

in 1993 that women who took vitamin E supplements for two years cut their risk of coronary artery disease in half compared to women who didn't take the supplements.[4]

• The well-known Cambridge Heart Antioxidant Study (CHAOS) looked at forty thousand men who already had heart disease. The study found that vitamin E kept their heart disease from getting worse. The men who took at least 400 IU of vitamin E a day cut their risk of having a nonfatal heart attack by an amazing 77 percent.[5]

• A long-term study of postmenopausal women showed that those who ate the most foods high in vitamin E (such as nuts, vegetable oils, and avocado) had strikingly less heart disease. That's without even taking vitamin E supplements.[6]

Vitamin E also makes your blood "thinner" in general, so it's less likely to clot where you don't want it to—in an artery leading to your heart or brain. In fact, vitamin E works almost as well as the anticoagulating drug warfarin (Coumadin®), but in a different way. Vitamin E prevents the tiny blood-clotting particles called platelets from clumping together. Of course, it also costs a lot less. (Vitamin E works so well to reduce your blood's ability to clot that you should stop taking it for a couple of weeks before any scheduled surgery.)

Now, what about vitamin C? The evidence here is also very solid, but I'll stick to just a couple of very strong pieces of recent research.

• If your blood levels of vitamin C are low to the point of deficiency, your risk of a heart attack is about 3.5 times greater than someone whose level is normal.[7]

In this day and age of fortified foods, how many people are really low in vitamin C? You'd be surprised—a recent study showed that overall, about 30 percent of the adult population is low on vitamin C, and more than 6 percent are outright deficient.[8] All these people are at greater risk from heart disease—as well as cancer, cataracts, and other problems that could be prevented by simple, safe, and very inexpensive vitamin supplements.

If you already have atherosclerosis, your chances of having a heart attack or an episode of unstable angina are much higher if you're also low on vitamin C. The vitamin C doesn't do anything to reduce the size of plaques, but it does keep them from rupturing and causing a blockage in the artery.[9]

As you can see, the evidence is strong. Recently, however, what I believe to be a misconception has arisen about vitamin C. In 1998, researchers reported that high doses of vitamin C seemed actually to cause free radical damage to the DNA in your cells. The antivitamin medical establishment and the media seized on this opportunity to undermine vitamin C. They took a single, very short research letter—not a full-fledged, peer-reviewed scientific study—with very tentative conclusions and made it sound as if taking a vitamin C supplement could have extremely negative consequences.[10]

What the media reports didn't tell you is that even an ordinary celery stalk contains compounds that can damage DNA. The media also didn't tell you that *too little* vitamin C is well-known to cause DNA damage.[11] That knowledge should get you to ask the critics, "With regard to protecting DNA, what is the optimal range of vitamin C?" I don't know what they'll say, but I know what I would: "It's whatever it was before that research letter was published."

Selenium

Selenium's role in preventing heart disease is sometimes overlooked. In fact, low selenium levels, like low vitamin C levels, are a serious risk factor for heart disease.[12]

Protecting Your Brain

Your brain has trillions of closely packed cells that communicate across cell membranes. Free radicals attack the membranes and damage the lines of communication, closing them down. Antioxidants can help keep these lines open and static free—so the best protection you can give your brain is to keep your antioxidant levels high. Huge amounts of research have been done in this area, and an awful lot of it points to antioxidants as a valuable way to prevent memory loss, Alzheimer's disease, and other cognition problems related to aging.

Let's see specifically how the antioxidant vitamins can protect your brain.

• In a recent study of retired people in Australia, the ones who took vitamin C supplements showed significantly less cognitive impairment—60 percent less. When the researchers added in dietary vitamin C, the number jumped to almost 70 percent less impairment.[13]

• A high intake of vitamin E can help ward off the annoying memory problems associated with aging. In a study of healthy older people age fifty to seventy-five, the people with the highest blood level of vitamin E did best on tests of memory. Why? Because vitamin E protects your brain cells—which are particularly high in fat—against the damaging effects of free radicals.[14]

• Vitamin E was just as effective as the drug selegiline in significantly slowing the progression of Alzheimer's disease—without the major expense of the drug.[15]

• Lipoic acid may play a part in preventing the cell damage that causes Alzheimer's disease—and may also help slow the damage if it does start. The research here is very promising.[16]

Valuable as vitamin E and vitamin C are for keeping your blood vessels clear of plaque, other vitanutrients, such as ginkgo biloba, are extremely valuable for cerebral circulation. I'll get to them later on, in Chapter 18.

Preventing Cancer

I have emphasized how valuable the eradication of cardiovascular disease is to extending your life span. I'm sure you've correctly guessed which other illness would, if eradicated, be second to heart disease. It is, of course, cancer.

Your chances of getting cancer go up as you age. Is that something you just have to accept? Absolutely not. You can take all sorts of positive steps to prevent cancer through vitanutrients. Indeed, vitamin C is proving to be one of the most powerful anticarcinogenic agents of all.[17]

I could write a whole book just discussing the many studies that prove the value of vitamin C against cancer. Let me just get right to the point instead: Vitamin C sharply reduces your chances of getting cancers of the stomach, esophagus, colon, bladder, cervix, uterus, and breast.[18] It probably protects you against many other cancers as well, but the evidence isn't as clear-cut on those.

There have been hundreds of positive studies showing that overall, the more vitamin E you get, the lower are your chances of getting cancer of any sort. To give you the idea, let's take a look at the most recent results from an ongoing research project called the Alpha-Tocopherol, Beta-Carotene Cancer Prevention Study (the ABC study for short). In 1998, the ABC study showed that vitamin E supplementation can protect against prostate cancer. First, the study showed that men over fifty who take just 50 IU of supplemental vitamin E have a 36 percent lower incidence of prostate cancer. Next, of the men who do get prostate cancer, taking vitamin E cuts their chance of dying from it by 41 percent.[19] Bear in mind that there are about one hundred thousand new cases of prostate cancer in the United States each year. Reducing its incidence by almost a third by using a vitanutrient that costs just a few pennies a day would have a major impact on national health care costs. (Another vitanutrient called lycopene also protects against prostate cancer. I'll discuss it in depth in Chapter 10.)

Alternative practitioners like myself have known for a long time that the trace mineral selenium helps prevent cancer. Our belief was vindicated by the results of a major study published in 1996. More than thirteen hundred patients were in the study, with half taking daily 200 mcg selenium supplements and half taking a placebo. At the end of the ten-year study, the patients who took selenium supplements had sharply lowered rates of some cancers. The selenium group had 63 percent fewer prostate cancers, 67 percent fewer esophageal cancers, 58 percent fewer colorectal cancers, and 46 percent fewer lung cancers. Overall, the selenium supplements reduced the number of cancers in the group by a third and cut cancer deaths in half.[20] The results of this important study were published in the *Journal of the American Medical Association*. Typically for mainstream medicine, an accompanying editorial was headlined "Selenium and cancer prevention: Promising results indicate further trials required."[21] As has often been the case with any vitanutrient approach to illness, the AMA has not made a recommendation and instead insists that more study is needed, but in the meantime many lives could be extended.

The protective effect of selenium against cancer has since been confirmed by a number of other studies. To take just one good example, a study of more than thirty-three thousand men showed that selenium reduces the risk of prostate cancer. Specifically, the risk of prostate cancer for men who took 200 mcg of selenium every day over a five-year period was one-third that of men who took a placebo instead.[22] The evidence is so powerful that I don't think I need to say anything more.

Vitanutrients in Perspective

So far I've told you about the effects of individual antioxidants in warding off cancer. In so doing I am party to the same mistake that mainstream advocates make when they insist that research to establish proof of value of nutritional agents has to be done one vitanutrient at a time. There's no question that antioxidants work as a team and that they should be given and tested as such.

Atkins Center patients at risk for a recurrence of cancer are routinely given an entire battery of antioxidants, not just one vitanutrient that's been shown to help. All our doctors are convinced that our recurrence rate is dramatically lower than that achieved by those treated in the conventional way with chemotherapy and/or radiation.

Saving Your Sight with Antioxidants

Another age-related problem affecting may people is loss of vision. The delicate structures of your eyes are particularly vulnerable to free radical damage, mostly because your eyes are exposed to a lot of ultraviolet light. The older you get, the more damage is done and the higher your risk of sight-robbing cataracts and macular degeneration becomes. By keeping your levels of vitamin C and vitamin E high, you can do a lot to avoid these problems.

In fact, taking vitamin E supplements could cut your risk of a cataract by half.[23] Even a regular one-a-day multivitamin supplement that contains only small amounts of vitamin E cuts your chances of a cataract by about 25 percent.[24]

If you think that's impressive, look at the statistics for vitamin C. Taking vitamin C supplements on a long-term basis could cut your risk of a cataract by 77 percent, according to a 1997 study of women who had been taking extra vitamin C for ten years or more.[25]

Given that about 12 percent of the annual Medicare budget goes for cataract surgery, here's another example of how taking vitanutrients saves not just your health but also your money.

Antioxidant vitamins and other antioxidant nutrients are also crucial for preventing macular degeneration, the leading cause of blindness among adults over fifty. Current projections are for some thirteen million cases among older Americans by 2030. As I'll explain in Chapter 10, many of these cases could be prevented by taking vitamin C and vitamin E along with supplements containing carotenoids such as lutein and zeaxanthin. Of course, eating plenty of the foods that contain these substances naturally, including dark green leafy vegetables such as kale, will also help.

Immunity and Antioxidants

As you've gotten older, you may have noticed that minor illnesses you once shook off easily now stay with you longer. Reduced immunity is part of the aging process, but there are active steps you can take through vitanutrients to keep your immune system functioning at peak capacity. This is so important for your ongoing health and longevity that I've devoted all of Chapter 15 to information on how to build your immunity.

Choosing Your Supplements

You'll need to take fairly high—but extremely safe—amounts of the antioxidant vitamins to get their protective effects. The benefits of vitamin E, for instance, show up only in daily doses of at least 50 IU and preferably much higher—at least 400 IU. There's no reasonable way you can eat enough foods high in vitamin E to get those amounts. Even a typical daily multivitamin supplement has only 30 IU. To get anywhere near levels that would do you some good, you'll have to take supplements.

Vitamin E supplements even in very large doses of more than 2,000 IU daily are perfectly safe for just about everybody. When you're choosing a vitamin E supplement, look for one that contains natural mixed tocopherols. That's the way vitamin E appears in nature, which means that's the way your body is designed to absorb it. To get the maximum benefit from your vitamin E capsules, take them with a meal. The fat in your food helps your body absorb the vitamin.

Today many manufacturers make vitamin E capsules with added selenium. This is a good, convenient way to be sure you're getting the best of both vitanutrients. In general, you need about 400 mcg a day to get the most protection from selenium.

Given that the RDA for vitamin C is a ridiculously low 60 mg, you might not think that anyone could really be deficient. (The RDA will probably be raised to between 100 and 200 mg in the near future—an improvement, but still far too low.) In fact, about a quarter of all Americans get less than 40 mg a day from their food.[26]

There is no better, cheaper, and more effective way to prevent most of the health problems I've just discussed than to give everyone the optimal dose of vitamin C every day. What would that be? My usual recommended range is 800 to 2,000 mg, but I don't hesitate to prescribe more for the many patients who report feeling better on higher dosages.

Because vitamin C is water soluble and quickly excreted, spread your dose out over the day. Taking it all at once will lead to a lot of wasted ascorbate.

Lipoic acid is another extremely safe vitanutrient. I usually recommend between 200 and 400 mg a day.

Now that you've got a good grasp of your first line of defense against free radical damage, let's move on to ways to enhance your body's other major defense system, the antioxidant enzymes. Here's where your increased vitamin and mineral intake pays off, because without these substances, your body can't make the enzymes efficiently.

9

The Antioxidant Enzymes

Humans are among the most long-lived of animals (only some kinds of turtles and perhaps a few whales outlive us). Humans also have very high levels of antioxidant enzymes, higher than just about any other animal. The link between long life and high levels of antioxidant enzymes is not coincidental. The antioxidant enzymes are a powerful force for longevity—and we'll learn all about them in this chapter. We'll also explore a couple of the most promising new age-defying antioxidants: coenzyme Q_{10} and melatonin.

SOD, Catalase, and Glutathione

The antioxidant enzyme superoxide dismutase, or SOD, works hand in hand with catalase and glutathione to quickly disarm the most dangerous free radicals. Here's how the two enzymes interact: When normal metabolism inside your mitochondria makes superoxide free radicals, SOD quickly converts them into oxygen and hydrogen peroxide. There's a problem with that, though. When a superoxide free radical meets hydrogen peroxide, it forms the very reactive free radical known as hydroxyl. Of all the free radicals, hydroxyl is the biggest vandal, the one that does the most damage in your body. You need to quench it instantly, as soon as it's produced. Unfortunately, your body doesn't make an enzyme that can quench the hydroxyl radical (although, as I'll discuss later in this chapter, you do have other defenses). That's where catalase comes in. Catalase grabs the hydrogen peroxide and breaks it up into oxygen and plain water before it can form a hydroxyl radical. The oxygen and water then get reused by your cells as part of normal metabolism.

Catalase has one big limitation: It works only in the watery parts of your cells. It can't protect the fatty parts of a cell, like the cell membrane, from lipid peroxides—the free radicals that are formed when hydrogen peroxide attacks lipids.

That's where glutathione comes in. Glutathione is the most abundant antioxidant enzyme in your body. It's everywhere—inside and outside of your cells, constantly patrolling your cells and looking for any molecules of hydrogen peroxide your catalase has missed. Glutathione also protects your cell membranes against lipid peroxidation. Simply put, lipid peroxidation happens whenever any free radical steals an electron from the delicate fatty membrane of a cell. Lipid peroxidation, like all free radical damage, is a chain reaction that keeps going until something—in this case, glutathione peroxidase—stops it. Without the glutathione, the damage would continue, weakening the cell membrane further and further until finally the cell is irretrievably damaged and dies. If the lipid peroxides are quenched quickly, however, your body can repair the cell membrane and get things working properly again.

Raising Your Enzyme Levels

Since your antioxidant enzymes are manufactured inside your cells by your body as you need them, is there anything you can do to raise their levels? Yes, at least to some degree.

Like all the proteins in your body, enzymes are assembled in your cells, following directions given by the DNA in the nucleus of every cell, from building blocks called amino acids. You also need vitamins such as vitamin C and the B vitamins and trace amounts of some minerals, such as copper, zinc, manganese, and iron, to help the proteins fit together properly.

If you give your cells enough of all the building blocks, they'll be able to put together the antioxidant enzymes just as quickly as you need them. Starve your cells of what they need, however, and the enzymes won't be assembled quickly enough. Even worse, without a regular supply of essential ingredients, your antioxidant enzymes could get out of balance. If you make enough SOD but not enough catalase, for instance, the all-important balance between the two is thrown off. They won't be able to work in tandem to protect you.

Think back to what I said earlier about amino acids as the building blocks of protein. Where do you get amino acids from? Your food. But not all foods are equal when it comes to aminos. To get what nutritionists call high-quality or complete protein, you need to eat animal foods such as meat, eggs, fish, and dairy products.

Eat Your Eggs

And of all those high-quality proteins, which one is the very best? If you've read my other books, you already know. For those of you who haven't yet, the answer is the egg. In fact, the egg is the standard nutritionists use to measure the quality of other proteins.

If eggs are such a good source of the essential amino acids, why does your conventional doctor tell you to eat them only occasionally? Because he or she thinks eggs raise your cholesterol level. As with so much of the other cholesterol misinformation you're given, this is the argument put forward by the American Heart Association. The AHA says you should take in only 300 mg a day of dietary cholesterol. Therefore, you shouldn't eat eggs, because one egg has about 215 mg of cholesterol (more than most other foods have for the same number of calories). As anyone who's ever read one of my books or heard one of my radio broadcasts knows, however, there's very little connection between the cholesterol you eat and the cholesterol in your blood. I could cite dozens of studies that show the opposite of the AHA position: that eating eggs actually improves your blood cholesterol profile. Here's just one good example. In a 1994 study, twenty-four adults added two eggs a day to their usual diets for six weeks. At the end of the period, their total cholesterol levels had increased by 4 percent. Their all-important HDL levels, however, were up a very desirable 10 percent.[1]

I'm glad to say that some members of the conventional medical world are finally starting to re-evaluate their position. In 1999, the National Institutes of Health funded a major study that showed that eating an egg a day doesn't increase the risk of heart disease or stroke for healthy adults.[2]

Many of the patients who first come to me at the Atkins Center have eliminated eggs from their diet, in the mistaken belief that they're doing something positive for their health. One of the first things I recommend to them is to start eating eggs again, at least two a day.

Enzyme Supplements

Because SOD and catalase are meant to exist within cells and are unstable inside the intestinal tract, you can't expect to take them as oral supplements and thereby boost your levels. A few manufacturers do make SOD tablets, but I don't think they will do much.

Oral glutathione supplements are used more often. Proponents feel that because glutathione is a tripeptide—a very short string of just three amino acids—it may avoid being broken down further by the digestive system. Instead, you can absorb it whole into the bloodstream. Most studies show rather disappointing elevations of serum glutathione after it is taken by mouth.

The far better way to raise your glutathione level is to raise your level of cysteine, an amino acid that's fundamental to manufacturing glutathione. We know that your blood levels of glutathione change in direct proportion to the amount of cysteine in your diet. The more cysteine you get, the more glutathione you make. And what's one of the very best dietary sources of cysteine? You guessed it—eggs. There are 146 mg of cysteine in one egg, most of it in the yolk. To raise glutathione levels more directly, I usually give my patients supplements of N-acetyl-cysteine, because the acetylated form leads to a higher glutathione level.

Vitamins and Minerals

To make all the antioxidant enzymes, you also need to have adequate supplies of the trace minerals zinc, manganese, copper, sulfur, and selenium. Manganese, copper, and zinc are particularly important for making SOD inside your mitochondria, where most of your free radicals are produced. Selenium and sulfur are crucial for forming glutathione. So, in addition to making sure you're getting enough high-quality protein every day, you need to get enough of the important trace minerals.

Finally, you need a goodly supply of vitamins, especially vitamin C and the B complex, to make the antioxidant enzymes. Vitamin C stimulates your body to produce extra catalase, for example. Without enough vitamin B_6 (pyridoxine), you can't make glutathione.

Coenzyme Q_{10}

Of all the vitanutrients I recommend for my patients, coenzyme Q_{10} (CoQ_{10}) is one of the most valuable. This essential vitanutrient is absolutely necessary for you to create energy in your mitochondria. No CoQ_{10}, no energy—it's as simple as that. CoQ_{10} is so important for your body that it's found in every single one of your cells.

When CoQ_{10} was discovered back in the late 1950s, researchers thought that its only function was helping in energy production. By the early 1960s, it was widely used in Japan to treat congestive heart failure. By the 1970s, Japanese researchers had learned ways to produce CoQ_{10} easily, and research into it really took off. By the 1980s, CoQ_{10} had become one of the five top-selling drugs in Japan. In the United States, the FDA has declared that CoQ_{10} is a dietary supplement with no real medical value. This means that despite its proven record for treating patients with cardiovascular disease, and despite its virtual absence of side effects, an American cardiologist is very unlikely ever to prescribe CoQ_{10} to a patient. Instead, you might be bombarded with dangerous drugs that simply mask the symptoms of your heart disease.

Let's look at how CoQ_{10} works in your body. CoQ_{10} is called a coenzyme because you need it to make at least three and possibly more of the enzymes you need to convert glucose and oxygen in your mitochondria into energy you can use. Once that energy is created, CoQ_{10} is also involved in the complex process of getting it out of your mitochondria and into the rest of your body.

CoQ_{10} also acts as an antioxidant inside your mitochondria, quenching superoxide radicals as they're formed.[3] Recent research, however, tells us that CoQ_{10} plays a bigger antioxidant role than we first realized. Because CoQ_{10} is everywhere in your body, and because it moves easily into and through your fatty cell membranes, it helps prevent damage to your cells from lipid peroxidation (free radical attacks on cell membranes). It also works synergistically with vitamin E, vitamin C, and lipoic acid to keep all those antioxidant vitanutrients working longer to protect you.[4]

You reach your peak production of CoQ_{10} at around age twenty. After that, your production gradually drops off; the drop gets faster as you pass forty. By the time you're eighty, you're naturally making only about 60 percent of your peak levels. At any age, though, your doctor may artificially lower your CoQ_{10} production to far below the optimal level. How? By prescribing cholesterol-lowering statin drugs such as Lovastatin®, simvistatin, and others. CoQ_{10} shares some of the same production pathways as cholesterol. When statin drugs block your production of cholesterol in your liver, they also block your production of CoQ_{10}. High-energy parts of your body, like your heart, need high concentrations of CoQ_{10}—in fact, the level of CoQ_{10} in your heart is twice that of other parts of your body. At the same time, CoQ_{10} is one of the most important antioxidants protecting your heart and arteries against athero-sclerosis.[5] If you've ever wondered why many studies show that the death rate from heart attacks for people who take statin drugs is still high, remember this: Their CoQ_{10} levels have been severely reduced.

To raise your CoQ_{10} level, you could eat foods that are high in it, such as sardines or beef liver, but you'd have to eat an awful lot of them for a dietary approach to have any real effect. Supplements are the way to go. As research continues, doctors keep learning that higher doses are more beneficial. By now the preventive dosage that I recommend is 50 to 100 mg daily. If you have any sort of health problem related to the heart, high blood pressure, metabolism, or energy level, you'll probably need more like 200 to 300 mg a day.

Melatonin: The Unsung Antioxidant

Melatonin has been in the news a lot lately for all sorts of reasons. This hormone is secreted by your pineal gland, a pea-sized structure found almost exactly in the center of your brain, and is used to regulate your body's twenty-four-hour clock. By now, you probably know that melatonin is a natural sleeping pill that can help reset your internal clock when it gets thrown off by jet lag or shift changes. You've probably also heard that melatonin can help boost your immune system and may even help prevent cancer.

What you may not know is that melatonin is also a very powerful antioxidant. Remember the dangerous hydroxyl radicals I mentioned a little earlier? Your antioxidant enzymes can't quench hydroxyl radicals, but melatonin can. Not only that, melatonin can stimulate your body to produce more of the other antioxidant enzymes I've just discussed. As with a lot of other hormones, you naturally make less melatonin as you get older. By the time you're fifty, you're making just a fraction of the melatonin you made as a teenager.

Melatonin is extremely important for protecting your cells—especially your brain cells—from the damaging effects of free radicals. According to Dr. Russell J. Reiter, the leading researcher in the field, melatonin mops up hydroxyl and peroxyl radicals "more efficiently than other known antioxidants."[6] In fact, melatonin is easily ten times as efficient as glutathione for neutralizing free radicals.[7]

Your brain is more vulnerable to free radical damage than just about any other part of your body. That's because nearly 50 percent of your brain by weight is fat. The hydroxyl radical is particularly damaging to fatty tissues, which means that your brain is the part of your body most likely to be damaged.

Fortunately, melatonin is especially good at protecting your brain because it can easily enter your brain cells to shield them from oxidative damage. That, in turn, may well protect you from Alzheimer's disease, memory problems, and other degenerative brain diseases.

Melatonin has a stimulatory effect on your antioxidant enzymes. Recent research shows that it boosts your production of SOD and glutathione. Because melatonin easily enters lipids, it easily enters the membranes of your cells. This helps to stabilize them and make them more resistant to oxidative attack.[8] Melatonin has been shown to be extremely safe. Doses of up to 6 grams have no toxic effects, although they will make you sleepy or slow your reaction time. In a recent clinical trial, fourteen hundred women in the Netherlands took 75 mg a day for up to four years with no ill effects.[9]

There are a few cautions for melatonin, though. Pregnant women should avoid it. So should women who are trying to get pregnant, because in high doses melatonin acts as a contraceptive. Because melatonin stimulates your immune system, questions may be raised about autoimmune diseases.

I've cited only some of the most recent breakthroughs in melatonin research. Nearly six thousand scientific articles have been published on melatonin. Even the august *New England Journal of Medicine* conceded in a 1997 article that melatonin has significant antioxidant abilities, can strengthen the immune system, can inhibit some tumors, and can induce sleep.[10]

This is a safe, inexpensive, and easily available supplement that provides outstanding antioxidant and antiaging protection. I recommend melatonin to all my patients over the age of fifty. Because melatonin is a hormone, the only way to raise your level of it is to take supplements. The usual starting dose for sleep is 3 mg at bedtime. When the immune-stimulating aspects of melatonin are being counted on, the dose could easily rise to 10 to 20 mg.

To avoid any problems from the sleepiness melatonin can cause, take the dose about half an hour before bedtime. As a bonus, you'll get a more refreshing night's sleep—and as you'll learn in Chapter 13, that can do more for you than you may know.

So far I've been discussing ways to raise your antioxidant levels through the use of vitanutrient supplements. The second prong of my approach to boosting your antioxidant levels is through a diet rich in nutrient-dense, high-antioxidant, low-carbohydrate foods. There are so many of these foods that I'll spend the next two chapters discussing them. After you read them, I'm certain you will conclude that the nutritional answer you are seeking will require both vitanutrients *and* a nutrient-dense diet.

10

Why You Need Carotenoids

Ever wonder why blueberries are blue or tomatoes are red? It's because plants, like people, need free radical protection. Botanists call the substances plants have evolved to protect themselves phytochemicals—literally, plant chemicals. Miraculously, the very same substances that protect plants and give them their characteristic colors and flavors are also the ones that protect people who eat those plants. Even more miraculously, the most colorful and protective plants are also the tastiest. As you'll discover in this chapter, vegetables and fruits are crammed with antioxidants and other substances that make all the difference to your health. If your diet is high in fresh vegetables and fruits, it's high in all kinds of protective vitanutrients. In addition, we can use supplements containing concentrated phytochemicals to help treat and prevent specific health problems.

The evidence in favor of phytochemicals from a diet rich in fruits and vegetables is overwhelming. We know from literally hundreds of recent studies that the antioxidants in fruits and vegetables slow brain aging, reduce your risk of just about every kind of cancer, protect your eyesight, and help prevent stroke and heart disease. Antioxidant phytochemicals also prevent diabetes and help reduce diabetic complications.

Researchers have already identified thousands of phytochemicals, and there are probably thousands more waiting to be discovered. This very promising area is getting a lot of research attention these days. I look forward to the day when we understand the phytochemicals and what they do so precisely that doctors prescribe foods instead of pharmaceuticals to treat and prevent most illnesses. Though it may not be in my lifetime, I firmly believe that in the century to come we will look back at our current dependence on drugs instead of diet in the same way we now look back at the nineteenth century's dependence on leeches and bloodletting—as crude, ineffective, and even harmful treatments based on ignorance.

Carotenoids

One of the most important clans within the phytochemical family, the carotenoids are a group of yellow-, orange-, and red-colored substances found in a wide variety of foods. As the name suggests, it's carotenoids, especially one called beta-carotene, that give carrots their orange color. Carotenoids also give squash and tomatoes their color, but many high-carotenoid foods, such as kale, are dark green. The carotenoids are still in there—they're just covered up by the green phytochemicals in the plant.

The carotenoid clan is enormous. So far, researchers have identified more than seven hundred different carotenoids, of which as many as fifty might be absorbed and used by the human body. We still don't know what, if anything, most of the carotenoids do for you if you eat them, because only fourteen or so have ever been found in human serum.[1] The relative handful of carotenoids that have been carefully studied, however, show that these phytochemicals provide powerhouse protection against free radical damage.

Some very interesting recent research also correlates carotenoids with protection from diabetes. Researchers at the federal Centers for Disease Control and Prevention looked at the levels of six major carotenoids—alpha-carotene, beta-carotene, cryptoxanthin, lutein, zeaxanthin, and lycopene—in more than one thousand people age forty to seventy-four with normal glucose tolerance. They then compared those levels to 277 people with impaired glucose tolerance and 148 people with newly diagnosed diabetes. Are you surprised to learn that the beta-carotene and lycopene concentrations were highest in the people with normal glucose tolerance, lower in those with impaired glucose tolerance, and lowest in the people with diabetes? I wasn't. This is yet another reason not to allow your sugar tolerance to become impaired.[2]

Let's look more closely at the carotenoids.

The Carotenes

In Chapter 8, I discussed the antioxidant vitamins, especially vitamin C and vitamin E. You may have wondered why I left out vitamin A. It's true that vitamin A is a valuable antioxidant. It's also true that one of vitamin A's main jobs in your body is preventing infection, so I often recommend supplements as part of the treatment for infections and wounds, lung disease, and other serious health problems. For basically healthy people, however, there's a better way to get all the vitamin A you need and also get extra antioxidant protection: consume carotenes.

Some of the vitamin A you get from your diet comes from

foods such as egg yolks, milk, and liver. The rest comes from plant foods that contain alpha- and beta-carotene, which your body easily converts into vitamin A in your small intestine and liver. (Some foods also contain gamma-carotene, but it doesn't seem to do much.) Only about 20 percent of the alpha-carotene you eat gets turned into vitamin A. The rest circulates in your system and enters your fatty tissues, where it is particularly good at mopping up the singlet oxygen radical and preventing lipid peroxidation—damage to the fatty cell membranes.[3]

Beta-carotene is much more abundant and much more active, by which I mean your body converts it very easily into vitamin A. But only about 40 percent of the beta-carotene that you eat turns into vitamin A. What happens to the rest? Like alpha-carotene, it circulates in your body and enters fatty tissues, where it acts as a very powerful antioxidant that protects you against heart disease and cancer. As a bonus, beta-carotene is also a major immune system booster.

Before I describe the exciting research into beta-carotene, let me just remind you that for optimal absorption and use of high-carotene foods, you need to eat them with some dietary fat. If you're on a low-fat diet, you won't absorb your carotenes particularly well. And here's another important point about the carotenes: They're carried around your system by your LDL cholesterol.[4] Yes, LDL cholesterol. Aren't you amazed to learn that "bad" cholesterol does good things for you? This is a good example of how your cholesterol can indeed be too low—you can't get the benefit of beta-carotene if you don't have enough LDL cholesterol to transport it around your body. In a good example of how your body has been created to be in balance, beta-carotene also raises your level of HDL cholesterol![5]

In general, people who have a lot of beta-carotene in their diets have lower risk of heart disease. An ongoing study of older Dutch adults showed exactly how much less. The study looked at the eating habits over four years of nearly five thousand healthy men and women between the ages of fifty-five and ninety-five. At the start of the study, none of the people had ever had a myocardial infarction (heart attack). At the end of the study, the people whose diets were highest in beta-carotene had a 45 percent reduction in their risk of a myocardial infarction compared to the people whose diets were lowest in beta-carotene. The protective effect of the beta-carotene was even higher among the smokers in the group—their risk of a heart attack was cut by 55 percent Among former smokers, the risk dropped by 68 percent.[6]

Despite the evidence in favor of beta-carotene, many conventional doctors don't recommend it for their patients. If they have any reasons beyond a negative reflex toward vitanutrients, they usually mention the results of the long-term Physicians' Health Study, which failed to show any benefit of beta-carotene in reducing the risk of heart disease or cancer.[7] (Or did it? I'll get to that a little later.) For now I'll just point out what I think is the big problem with that study: The doctors involved took only 83,000 IU every other day, but 41,500 IU a day is just barely enough to have any positive effect.

Many researchers believe that the optimal amount for cancer prevention is at least 70,000 IU a day. Getting that much a day from food is difficult—you'd have to eat about four cups of cooked carrots! The best way to be sure you're getting enough beta-carotene protection is through supplements.

Beta-carotene is one of the safest of all vitanutrients. It would be very difficult to overdose on it, even if you take 250,000 IU a day for months. At worst, your skin may temporarily turn a harmless orange color (the color fades away if you cut back your dose).[8] For patients with heart disease, the beta-carotene dose I usually prescribe is 90,000 IU a day.

Why does beta-carotene work so well against heart disease? Like other antioxidants such as vitamin C and vitamin E, beta-carotene keeps LDL cholesterol from oxidizing.

Despite some recent bad publicity, beta-carotene is also very effective in the fight against cancer, both preventing it and treating it. Before I go any farther in explaining why it helps, let's take a look at that bad publicity and see what was really going on.

In 1996, the Beta Carotene and Retinol Efficacy Trial study, better known as the CARET study, showed that taking beta-carotene supplements actually increased the rates of lung cancer in smokers.[9] The medical establishment seized on this study and the effect was to cast doubt on the whole idea of vitanutrients. As a result, a lot of people got the mistaken idea that beta-carotene causes all sorts of cancer in everyone.

Not so. The people in the study were all smokers, former smokers, or asbestos workers—people already at very high risk for lung cancer. Only the asbestos workers and the people who continued to smoke had an increased risk of lung cancer; the former smokers had a slightly *reduced* risk.

Despite the results of the CARET study, we know from a number of other positive studies that among nonsmokers, beta-carotene truly does have a positive effect on the lungs, protecting them not only against cancer but also against chronic pulmonary obstructive disease, including asthma, bronchitis, and emphysema.

What conclusions can we draw from all this? First, if you smoke, stop. Second, if my words, for some strange reason, don't result in your automatically quitting, then at least start eating high-antioxidant foods and supplement them with full-spectrum natural carotenoids rather than with synthetic beta-carotene.

Smoker or not, eating foods rich in carotenoids (as opposed to taking supplements) could do a lot to protect you against cancer of all sorts, including lung cancer.[10] As with heart disease, people who eat a lot of foods rich in beta-carotene, such as spinach, kale, and squash, have a reduced risk of cancer. I don't have room to discuss every study that shows how effective dietary beta-carotene is for cancer prevention, but almost all of them are attributed to full-spectrum carotenoids being taken as food. To look at just one excellent recent example, a Swedish study of postmenopausal women showed that a diet rich in beta-carotene appears to lower the risk of breast cancer. And the longer the women had been eating a high-beta-carotene diet, the better protected they were.[11]

When it comes to prostate cancer, however, supplements of beta-carotene may make a big difference. Remember the Physicians' Health Study that supposedly showed no cancer prevention benefit from beta-carotene? Researchers have been looking at the results a little more closely recently, and they're starting to backpedal. Among the twenty-two thousand male doctors taking part in the study, half took beta-carotene supplements in addition to their normal diets. Overall, the doctors who didn't eat many fruits and vegetables had low blood levels of beta-carotene—and were one-third more likely to develop prostate cancer. The men who took the beta-carotene supplements, however, were 36 percent less likely to develop prostate cancer, even if they skipped their fruits and vegetables. In this instance, the beta-carotene supplements seem to have made up for the lack of dietary carotenoids.[12]

The antioxidant power of beta-carotene is one way it fights cancer. Another way that beta-carotene helps cancer patients is by keeping their cells communicating properly. Many carcinogens disrupt cell-to-cell communications. That lets the cancer cells get a foothold before your immune system realizes it and can react. Beta-carotene helps keep the lines of communication—technically, the gap junctions—open. Even after cancer has started, restoring gap junction communication with extra beta-carotene may help reverse the process.[13]

My first mentor in the treatment of cancer was the late Dr. Hans Nieper of Hannover, Germany. Dr. Nieper was world-famous for the number of cancer survivors he had created. A mainstay of his therapy was beta-carotene, always given in doses high enough to produce a harmless yellowing of the palms of his patients. Nieper taught me that beta-carotene helps activate the thymus gland, one of your body's most important sources of immune protection. Beta-carotene also inactivates our own suppressor cells, the lymphocytes that turn off our immune responses.[14] Dr. Nieper's brilliant work was confirmed for me again when I read that researchers recently showed that beta-carotene also stimulates the activity of your natural killer cells. These are the immune cells that destroy cancerous cells and that are considered by researchers to be the white blood cells most involved in fighting cancer.[15]

Overall, beta-carotene is an excellent way to stimulate your immune system to fight off viruses and infections.[16] In fact, I often prescribe beta-carotene for my patients with chronic viral infections. Some of the beta-carotene is converted to vitamin A, which enhances immunity, but the beta-carotene also seems to help independent of its vitamin A activity.

Lycopene

Of all the carotenoids, lycopene is the one that's most effective for neutralizing the damaging singlet oxygen free radical.[17] Lycopene is the phytochemical that makes tomatoes red. Small amounts of lycopene are also found in watermelon and pink grapefruit, but for dietary lycopene, tomatoes are pretty much the only option. Of these, tomato juice and puree are the best choices.

Much of the recent research suggests that some of the benefits we once attributed to beta-carotene actually come from lycopene. In fact, lycopene offers more cancer protection than beta-carotene—perhaps as much as ten times more. It also offers more protection against LDL cholesterol oxidation, so lycopene is very good for protecting your arteries and heart against plaque formation. One of the interesting things about lycopene is that your body doesn't convert any of it to vitamin A.

You probably began hearing about lycopene back in 1995, when reports that it helps prevent prostate cancer first came out. That first study showed that men who eat at least ten servings a week of tomato-based foods are up to 45 percent less likely to develop prostate cancer.[18] And among men who do develop prostate cancer, treatment with lycopene may decrease tumor size and make the cancer less aggressive.[19]

Interestingly, the original study showed that these men's most common source of lycopene was tomato sauce. Like beta-carotene, lycopene can be absorbed into your body only if you eat it with some dietary fat. It's also best absorbed if it has been heated to release the lycopene from within the tomato cells.

Since that first announcement, lycopene has been shown to help prevent other cancers as well, including cancers of the lung, stomach, colon, and breast. In fact, eating a lot of lycopene seems to reduce your overall risk of cancer by about 40 percent.[20] To give you just one more specific example of how lycopene prevents cancer, smokers with low lycopene levels have four times more lung cancer than those with the highest levels.[21]

Lycopene's value isn't limited to cancer. A major recent European study compared the lycopene levels of men who had just had a first heart attack to those of men who were healthy. The ones who had the highest lycopene levels were half as likely to have a heart attack as those with the lowest levels.[22]

The latest research on lycopene suggests that it may well have a positive effect on your immune system. In a small study involving ten women, the ones who ate tomato puree every day for twenty-one days had higher blood levels of lycopene than the women who ate a tomato-free diet. The white blood cells of the tomato eaters were much more resistant to oxidative damage—anywhere from 33 to 42 percent more.[23] Even though this study was small, its results are important because it ties in the improvements in lycopene levels to something of known clinical significance for strengthening your immune system.

From my perspective, the problem with dietary lycopene is that it's valuable only if it's been processed. That's not bad in itself. The real problem comes from finding a way to eat two servings a day of tomato sauce or tomato paste that doesn't also involve a lot of carbohydrates like spaghetti. Those who need to have a major reduction in their carbohydrates should take a look at Table 21.4, which lists the carbohydrate-to-lycopene ratio of various foods. Select the foods that give you the best ratio, such as tomato puree or tomato soup. Even so, these foods tend to be high in carbohydrates, which is why many of my patients prefer to take lycopene in supplement form.

Lutein and Zeaxanthin

Among people over fifty, the leading cause of blindness is age-related macular degeneration (AMD), or loss of central vision. About thirteen million Americans have AMD, and nearly 25 percent of people over sixty-five have at least early signs of it. About three hundred thousand people go blind from AMD every year.

Well over half of all AMD cases could be avoided through two simple steps: stop smoking and eat foods high in the carotenes lutein and zeaxanthin. Smokers are two and a half times as likely to develop AMD as nonsmokers.[24]

Because your eyes are exposed to sunshine all the time, their tissues need to be very high in antioxidants to prevent damage caused by blue and ultraviolet light. Lutein and zeaxanthin are yellow—they give foods such as corn their color. These two carotenes are concentrated in your macula, the most sensitive area of the light-gathering retina at the back of your eye. Logic suggests they must be there for a purpose. Well, of course, they are. They form a yellowish deposit there that absorbs blue light, keeping it from generating damaging free radicals.

I could make a strong case for calling macular degeneration a vitamin deficiency disease, just like scurvy.[25] The only difference is that macular degeneration takes decades to show up. The best way to protect your eyes is by eating a diet rich in lutein and zeaxanthin. Lutein is found most abundantly in dark green leafy vegetables such as kale and spinach. Zeaxanthin is less abundant in foods but is found in yellow foods such as corn and orange peppers. Your body also converts some lutein into zeaxanthin. According to a recent study, people who ate the most foods rich in lutein and zeaxanthin had a 43 percent lower risk of developing AMD than those who ate the lowest amounts of these foods.[26]

What often gets left out of discussions of dietary ways to prevent AMD is the fact that egg yolks are the very best source of lutein and zeaxanthin. In fact, egg yolks contain higher concentrations of these carotenes than any other food.[27] Can you just imagine how much macular degeneration could have been prevented if egg yolks hadn't been seen as a dietary enemy for so long? Now you know how repulsed I am every time I see a hotel breakfast menu indicating that an egg-white omelette is a "healthy" choice—that you can get for an extra fifty cents. Next time you see that, think of me, think of your eyesight, and order a spinach omelette. See if you can get the waiter to throw in some leftover egg yolks from the AHA-victimized egg white devotees.

Macular degeneration can't be cured, but it can be slowed and even reversed a bit with vitanutrients. In one experiment, 102 people with macular degeneration took daily supplements of vitamin C, vitamin E, beta-carotene, and selenium. In 60 percent of the cases, deterioration of the macula stopped or improved.[28] If the program had included lutein and zeaxanthin supplements, I believe it would have worked for even more of the patients. At the Atkins Center we use such a combination of vitanutrients to treat AMD. The primary carotenoid supplement is 6 to 10 mg of lutein daily.

Olestra Alert!

Our fatphobic society has embraced olestra, an artificial, zero-calorie fat substitute also known as Olean. Snack foods containing olestra are now found on supermarket shelves everywhere. The FDA approved this product, although it did insist that Proctor & Gamble, the manufacturers, add vitamins A, D, E, and K to it. Why add the vitamins? Olestra is a fatty substance made from sugar and vegetable oil. It passes right through you without being digested, which means it binds up these crucial fat-soluble vitamins and carries them out of your body.

What the FDA didn't seem to appreciate is the way olestra also removes carotenoids. According to famed Harvard epidemiologist Meir J. Stampfer, people who eat just three small olestra-based snacks a week could expect at least a 10 percent drop in their carotenoid levels. In real terms, Stampfer projected that could mean thirty-two thousand additional deaths from cancer and heart disease each year.[29] You already know you should stay away from junk food of all sorts. Don't be snookered by advertising and the medical establishment into thinking that junk food made with olestra is somehow automatically safe to eat—or that healthful food made with it might not be turned into junk food

The Atkins Rx for Carotene Supplements

As I discussed above, there's a chance that taking synthetic beta-carotene supplements alone could trigger cancer in some people. I much prefer to have my patients take natural mixed-carotene supplements. These supplements contain all the carotenes, not just beta-carotene, so you get the complete antioxidant protection package. For basically healthy people, I suggest at least 10,000 IU daily and preferably more—up to 25,000 IU. Supplements made from an alga called *Dunaliella salina* or from whole-food concentrates provide the best mix of all the carotenes. And if you find a product that also brings in lutein, zeaxanthin, and lycopene, you've gotten the most out of this chapter.

Next we'll turn to the other major group of dietary antioxidants, the bioflavonoids.

11

The Benefits of Bioflavonoids

You know that foods like broccoli and kale are good for you, but do you know why? These foods, and many others, are crammed with health-giving bioflavonoids, phytochemicals that go by complicated names like anthocyanosides, sulforaphane, and resveratrol. Bioflavonoids are the completely natural chemicals that give these foods their characteristic colors and flavors. So far, researchers have discovered more than a thousand bioflavonoids in foods we commonly eat. Coincidentally (although if you're of a spiritual bent, you might not see it as a coincidence), some of the bioflavonoids in foods also happen to be excellent for treating and preventing common health problems.

Let's forget about the terminology and get straight to the benefits of bioflavonoids. Because all fruits and vegetables contain a number of phytochemicals with overlapping effects, I'm going to simplify things a bit by focusing just on the bioflavonoids I and those wonderful scientists who make discoveries have found most useful.

Green Tea: Antioxidants in a Cup

Tea is the most widely consumed beverage in the world, after plain water. It's also the most healthful thing you can drink, perhaps including plain water. What fascinates me about tea is that it seems to help just about everything, from cancer to cavities.

Ounce for ounce, green tea, made from the leaves of the plant *Camellia sinenis*, contains more antioxidant compounds and other phytochemicals than any other food or beverage. Black tea, the kind most Americans drink, has been processed somewhat and has fewer flavonoids. Even so, black tea has almost as much health-giving value as green tea.[1]

What exactly is in tea? Both black and green tea contain polyphenols, a group of chemical compounds that are powerful antioxidants and have other useful health effects. In general, people who drink a lot of tea are healthier overall. In part, that could be because people who drink a lot of tea don't drink a lot of other things, like sugary soft drinks or alcohol, that are certainly bad for you. Evidence shows, however, that there's more to the story than that.

Green tea is a valuable cancer preventive. A study in Shanghai, China, where green tea is a favorite beverage, showed that regular tea drinkers had a 50 percent lower risk of esophageal cancer.[2] A number of studies show a similar protective effect against other cancers, including cancers of the colon, breast, lung, stomach, and skin.[3] The protective effect is greatest if you don't smoke or drink alcohol. Even so, the antitumor effect of green tea could help explain a puzzling paradox: Even though many Japanese smoke cigarettes, the lung cancer rate in Japan is surprisingly low. The reason could well be their high tea consumption—six cups a day or more is typical in Japan.

How do the bioflavonoids in tea help you? The main effect seems to come from a group of substances called catechins. Four catechins are found abundantly in green tea. The one called epigallocatechin-3-gallate (EGCG) seems to be the most exciting of all, because is has a powerful anticancer action—without side effects.[4] The EGCG probably works by inhibiting the action of an enzyme needed for cell growth. EGCG doesn't affect healthy cells, but it shuts down the enzyme in cancerous cells. Instead of continuing to reproduce wildly, the cancer cells die.[5]

Your Heart Benefits, Too

The antioxidant flavonoids in tea are also a great way to protect your heart. In fact, some of the flavonoids in green tea are up to twenty-five times as powerful as vitamin E and one hundred times as powerful as vitamin C in quenching free radicals.[6] With that sort of antioxidant protection, it's not surprising that people who drink one or more cups of tea a day have a 46 percent reduction in heart attack risk compared to non–tea drinkers.[7]

The protection extends to your stroke risk as well. The famous Zutphen study, which looked at the stroke risk among a group of more than five hundred Dutch men over a fifteen-year period, showed that the men who had the highest intake of flavonoids had the lowest risk of stroke. The main source of flavonoids in their diet—70 percent of the total—turned out to be black tea. The men who drank more than four cups of tea a day had a two-thirds lower risk of stroke than men who drank fewer than two to three cups a day.[8]

The antioxidant power of tea isn't the only thing that helps fend off heart attacks and strokes. Tea also acts as a mild anticoagulant that keeps your platelets from clumping up and making an artery-blocking clot.

More Benefits of Tea

I think one of the most promising areas of green tea research right now is in treating arthritis. The antioxidant power of the green tea's polyphenols blocks the pathway of the Cox-2 enzyme, which is a major cause of the inflammation and pain of arthritis. The polyphenols work in very much the same way as the new, heavily advertised antiarthritis drugs such as Celebrex®, except that the tea doesn't have the risk of potentially dangerous side effects—or a high cost.[9]

Tea also has a strong antibacterial effect. Drinking a cup of tea after a meal helps prevent cavities and gum disease because the polyphenols kill the bacteria that cause these diseases. We know from other research that there's a high correlation between gum disease and heart disease. Could that be one reason for the lower heart risk among tea drinkers?

In the test tube, green tea also fights one of today's major medical problems: antibiotic-resistant bacteria. Because of the thoughtless, pointless overprescribing of unnecessary antibiotics by conventional doctors, today we are faced with the very serious problem of dangerous bacteria that have become drug resistant. These bacteria can cause severe, even fatal infections that don't respond to drug treatment. Recent research shows that extracts of green tea may actually reverse penicillin resistance in some strains of drug-resistant bacteria. In fact, the tea seems to act synergistically with the antibiotics to make them even more potent.[10]

Of course, this work is still in the experimental stage, but I find it quite interesting. I very rarely prescribe antibiotics for my patients. Unfortunately, there are some illnesses, such as Lyme disease and the new stealth bacteria epidemic, that can't really be treated with vitanutrients and diet alone. For those unusual times when I do have to prescribe antibiotics, I always accompany them with restoration doses of beneficial bacteria and natural substances that inhibit the growth of antibiotics' number-one complication—yeast overgrowth.

The amount of polyphenols and other flavonoids in a cup of freshly made tea can vary enormously. Depending on the tea variety and how it was processed and brewed, there can be anywhere from 50 to 400 mg of polyphenols in a single cup. The polyphenol content of green tea is much higher than in black tea. I strongly recommend choosing green tea over black tea, but any tea is better than none.

How much green tea is enough to prevent health problems? That's a good question. Some studies suggest that you need to sip at least six cups a day. In the Shanghai study of esophageal cancer, though, the positive effect of green tea was noted even in people who drank only a cup a day.

I enjoy sipping a cup of tea, green or black, but to make sure my patients get the same amount of the polyphenols every time, I recommend supplements of green tea extract. Choose a brand that's standardized to contain 35 percent EGCG.

Quercetin

Quercetin is one of my favorite flavonoids, and much research confirms its premier status. At the Atkins Center we use it as a major component of our treatment for allergies, because quercetin naturally blocks some of the histamines your body produces in response to pollen and other allergens. The same blocking effect also works to make quercetin quite effective for treating inflammation of any sort, including arthritis. Quercetin is also of significant help in treating heart disease and cancer.

Like most of the flavonoids, quercetin acts as an anticoagulant that keeps your blood from clotting. It also protects LDL cholesterol from oxidation, which prevents plaque buildup. Both effects, of course, help lower your risk of a heart attack or stroke.

Quercetin is considered the single most powerful antioxidant flavonoid. A new flavonoid called DHQ (dihydroquercetin), which may outstrip quercetin fourfold, is the one we're studying at the Atkins Center. Both are especially helpful for scavenging the peroxyl radical and preventing lipid peroxidation (oxidative damage to fatty parts of the body, such as cell membranes).[11]

As a cancer treatment and preventive, quercetin shows a lot of promise. In humans, quercetin is a valuable treatment for leukemia and breast cancer. It may well be valuable for other cancers, including colon cancer, ovarian cancer, and others—but so far, the studies are only in animals.

The best dietary source of quercetin is the humble onion. Eating one big onion—raw or cooked—is enough to raise your quercetin level noticeably within a few hours. Apples also contain quercetin, but your body can't absorb it as well. Other dietary sources include tomatoes and broccoli, and there's even some quercetin in green tea. The amounts of quercetin you need to help prevent disease, however, are fairly substantial. To get enough really to make a difference, you'll almost certainly need to take supplements. I usually recommend anywhere from 500 to 1,000 mg a day as a basic preventive against heart disease and cancer. In the case of DHQ, the equivalent dose is 200 to 500 mg daily.

Citrus flavonoids such as rutin, naringin, and hesperidin

are closely related to quercetin. For that reason, I use the citrus flavonoids as part of my treatment for patients with hay fever and other allergies. For other uses, however, citrus flavonoid supplements aren't that effective—I prefer to use quercetin. If you want to try them, I suggest taking mixed flavonoids from a reliable manufacturer that specifies the amounts of each substance in the supplement.

A word of caution here: Naringinen, a citrus bioflavonoid found in grapefruit juice, can interact badly with certain drugs, particularly beta-blockers used to treat high blood pressure and angina. If you are still taking drugs such as felodipine (Plendil®) or nifedipine (Procardia®), don't drink grapefruit juice or take citrus bioflavonoids.*

Garlic

Pungent foods like onions and garlic are strong tasting because they're full of valuable bioflavonoids. Garlic is so crammed with complex flavonoids, vitamins, and minerals such as selenium and zinc that it's very hard to say specifically which substance gives it the most antioxidant power. The overall effect, however, is awesome. I could write a whole chapter on garlic's benefits, but I'll focus here just on garlic's antioxidant power.

Garlic reduces your risk of heart disease. It lowers cholesterol and triglycerides, lowers blood pressure, and acts as a natural anticoagulant in your blood.

The primary protection for your heart comes from garlic's antioxidant capacity. Garlic has been shown in a number of studies to reduce LDL oxidation and prevent arteriosclerosis.

*For information on nutritional alternatives to taking beta-blocker drugs, see *Dr. Atkins' Vita-Nutrient Solution.*

In fact, in Germany, garlic supplements are routinely pre-scribed to treat arteriosclerosis. They work extremely well. A recent study in Germany showed that taking garlic supple-ments makes your aorta, the main artery carrying blood from your heart to the rest of your body, more flexible. Your aorta naturally gets stiffer as you age, but the aortas of men in the study who took garlic supplements were on average 15 percent more elastic than those of other men in their age group.[12] An-other German study suggests that garlic not only prevents the buildup of plaque in arteries but may even reduce it. Patients who took garlic supplements markedly slowed their rates of plaque buildup compared to the control group.[13]

Many, many laboratory experiments in the test tube and with animals show that garlic is a potent inhibitor of cancer. We don't have anywhere near as much evidence that it works in people, but I feel confident that the proof will soon be found. The research is extremely promising. For example, a com-pound found in aged garlic has been shown to dramatically diminish the growth of human prostate cancer cells, at least in the lab. A sulfur compound that forms as garlic ages seems to be the active ingredient.[14]

Is fresh garlic better than aged garlic extract? Well, I like both. It's possible that the extract has greater anticancer bene-fits, but the more garlic you take in any form, the more benefit you get. For some people, it's much easier to swallow odorless, tasteless garlic capsules than to eat a lot of garlic. Personally, I love garlic in my food. If you use the extract, I suggest a daily dose of 1,000 mg.

OPCs: Powerful Antioxidants

Here's another example of valuable flavonoids found in foods—but in such low concentrations that you need to take supplements to get the full benefit. The oligomeric proanthocyani-dins—OPCs for short—are a group of flavonoids found in grape seeds, berries, and the bark of some pine tree species. No matter where they come from, OPCs are powerful antioxidants—as much as fifty times more potent than equivalent amounts of vitamins C and E. They're extremely good at scavenging hydroxyl free radicals and preventing lipid peroxidation.

I find OPCs most useful for improving circulation. These substances are particularly valuable for building up the integrity of blood vessel walls. This is crucial. You need strong capillaries (tiny blood vessels) to carry blood to all your cells. Good capillary circulation is especially important for the health of your brain, eyes, hands, and feet. OPCs restore and maintain good circulation, and also reduce easy bruising, varicose veins, and other circulatory problems. They're helpful too for treating eye problems such as macular degeneration and diabetic retinopathy.

One popular way to get your proanthocyanidins is through extracts made from the bark of pine trees. A patented version of pine-bark extract called Pycnogenol is widely sold as a dietary supplement. The OPC concentration in Pycnogenol is about 85 percent. For a slightly higher (up to 95 percent) concentration of OPCs, try supplements made from grape seeds. These have the advantage of being less expensive as well. In general, I recommend taking a daily dose of 100 to 200 mg, measured as 95 percent OPCs.

Anthocyanocides, the OPCs found in blueberries, bilberries (a very close Scandinavian cousin of blueberries), blackberries, red cherries, and strawberries, are also good antioxidants. Bilberries contain by far the highest concentration of anthocyanocides, which is why they're used in supplements to the exclusion of all the other berries. Bilberry supplements are very helpful for protecting your vision, especially your night vision, as you age. If you've noticed that driving at night is getting more difficult, taking bilberry supplements might be very helpful. Bilberry has also been shown to be an effective treatment for macular degeneration and diabetic retinopathy.

What About Wine?

People who drink moderate amounts of red wine—one to three glasses a day—have less heart disease and cancer and live longer than nondrinkers. Recent research suggests that it's an OPC called resveratrol in the wine, not the alcohol, that does the trick. Resveratrol is found in grape skins, so you get some whenever you drink grape juice, whether or not it's fermented. Relatively speaking, resveratrol isn't that potent an antioxidant—it's only about half as effective as OPCs. If you already habitually drink a glass or two of wine each day, you're getting some extra antioxidant protection and there's no reason to stop. If you don't usually have wine, though, there's no need to start drinking it. In fact, if you have any sort of blood sugar problem, it's best to avoid alcohol in any form. You can take resveratrol supplements, but you'll get the same or greater benefit from grape seed supplements.

Ginkgo Biloba

Ginkgo biloba, an extract made from the leaves of the ginkgo tree, is one of the most important vitanutrients for inhibiting brain aging. I'll be discussing it in that capacity much more in Chapter 18 on brain aging.

The antioxidant flavones that make ginkgo work so well in your brain also help other aspects of your health. I believe it's one of the most important of all the plant-based medicines. I'm hardly alone in this. In Europe, where ginkgo has been a part of standard medicine for years, it makes up nearly 1 percent of all pharmaceutical purchases. Total annual sales of ginkgo products worldwide are now over $1 billion.

More than three hundred studies demonstrate that ginkgo improves the flow of blood through your circulatory system. As I'll discuss in Chapter 18, it's particularly good for improving the flow of blood to your brain, where it protects your brain cells from oxidative stress and improves memory and mental function.

Elsewhere in your body, improved circulation can help treat a wide range of problems. Ginkgo supplements help improve male sexual function, stabilize irregular heart rhythms, and relieve the discomfort of intermittent claudication, a circulatory disorder in the legs. By improving circulation through the tiny blood vessels of your eyes, ginkgo also helps protect you against problems such as macular degeneration and cataracts. Similarly, improving circulation to the ears helps problems such as hearing loss and tinnitus.

Ginkgo biloba is also particularly good for cleaning up the damaging superoxide radical.

Not only is ginkgo biloba extremely effective, it's extremely safe. Even very large doses over a long period are unlikely to have any harmful effects. For patients over forty, I usually advise taking at least 60 mg three times a day. Choose a ginkgo supplement that has been standardized to contain 24 percent ginkgo flavonoids and 6 percent terpenes.

Eat Your Vegetables!

You can't open a magazine or newspaper today without reading something about the health-giving qualities of vegetables.

You're constantly being urged to eat more cruciferous vegetables, like cabbage, kale, and brussels sprouts, and more dark-green leafy vegetables, like Swiss chard and beet greens. Why? To give just one good reason, eating cruciferous vegetables could sharply reduce your chances of colon cancer.[15] These plants are full of fiber, vitamins, and minerals, of course, but they're also full of a wide range of flavonoids—and it's the flavonoids that provide a lot of the protection.

As I've discussed in this chapter, we know what a lot of those flavonoids do—and we also know that about 30 percent of the antioxidant activity of these foods comes from flavonoids that haven't been identified yet. (And those that you read about in this chapter are merely a sample of what *is* known.) That's why you're always being told to eat a variety of vegetables. You get the benefit of all the flavonoids, including the ones that don't have names. And as I've stressed over and over, keeping your antioxidant level high is your best protection against cancer, heart disease, and all the other diseases that are supposedly a "normal" part of growing older.

Not all vegetables are created equal, however. You need to balance the total antioxidant value of a vegetable against its carbohydrate content, and some of you need to do so more than others. Sweet potatoes, for instance, are a great source of beta-carotene, minerals, and flavonoids, but they're also very high in carbohydrates. That means that those of you who have problems with weight, blood sugar, triglycerides, or high blood pressure might be better off looking for a different vegetable. To help you decide which vegetables give you the most flavonoids for the least carbohydrates, see the tables in Chapter 21.

Similarly, fruits are full of good nutrition but also have a lot of both fructose and glucose. Here too you need to balance antioxidants against carbohydrates—and simple sugars. As you'll learn in Chapter 21, most fruits—with the exception of berries—are far too high in sugar for the flavonoids you get from them.

Learning how to achieve that balance of carbohydrate/flavonoid content is such a central part of your age-defying diet that all of Chapter 21 is devoted to discussing it.

Going beyond antioxidants in all their variety, there are major steps we can take to slow or even reverse the aging process. Techniques such as hormone optimization and chelation therapy hold out tremendous promise to all who would defy aging. Let me tell you about them.

PART IV

Techniques to Defy Aging

The age-defying techniques I use at the Atkins Center start with diet but go far beyond it. Among the techniques I'll discuss in this part are:

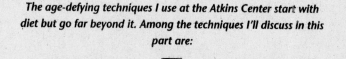

Hormone optimizing to restore your hormones to more youthful levels—a subject so important that I have devoted two long chapters to it.

Improving your immunity through dietary changes and vitanutrients such as vitamin A, zinc, and garlic.

Detoxifying your body through chelation therapy and by restoring your intestinal tract to a desirable balance.

Exercising for a healthier heart, better glucose tolerance, lower blood pressure, and weight loss.

Boosting your brain power with vitanutrients such as ginkgo biloba.

12

Reverse Declining Hormone Levels

You've probably noticed the impressive proliferation of "antiaging" clinics throughout the United States. A quick glance at their advertisements and brochures tells you that hormones are one of the mainstays of their treatment programs. The clinics promise to restore your hormones back to their levels when you were a youthful person in the prime of life. After looking at the brochure, your reaction might well be, "Makes sense, but it sounds too good to be true."

I agree. It does make sense, because the logic behind hormone restoration is supported by reams of scientific data. If done properly, hormone optimization or rebalancing (terms I prefer over "hormone restoration") is one of the well-established mainstays of age-defying medicine.

When it comes to the "too good to be true" part, that simply depends on "if done properly." That's crucial to success in hormone optimization. Doing it properly involves a thorough understanding of the interrelationships of all our hormones and an evidence-based system for knowing whether your hormonal levels—and I'm talking about *all* of them—are, in fact, at your individual optimal points.

What Hormones Do

Your body is an intricate living machine. Keeping all that complexity balanced and under control is the job of your hormones—powerful messenger chemicals made by your endocrine glands (your adrenal glands, ovaries or testicles, thyroid, parathyroids, pineal gland, pituitary gland, and pancreas) and sent into circulation in your bloodstream. Hormones regulate every aspect of your body's functions, from your blood pressure to your body temperature to your sex drive.

From birth until old age, much of what distinguishes you from everyone else is the relative preponderance of one hormone over another. But as we age, we all experience declines in virtually every hormone, some declining faster than others. Your production of hormones can decline quite rapidly as you age.

With the steady drop in your hormone levels come the symptoms of aging. What happens then? Your body gets weaker. You lose muscle mass and muscle tone, your bones become brittle, your blood vessels weaken, and you become less resistant to infection. Hormone decline also affects your mind. You become less alert, you get more anxious or depressed, you have trouble with short-term memory, and you may have trouble sleeping soundly. Your libido declines and you tire easily.

As your natural output of hormones inexorably declines, must your health and life span decline as well? Absolutely not. In the first place, our twentieth-century scientists have showed us ways to slow down the decline in most of these hormones.

When slowing the decline isn't enough and your body is still no longer making the hormones in sufficient quantity, we can safely replace them with hormone supplements. Scientists have shown us how we can do this safely and restore your hormone levels to the peaks you experienced when you were thirty.

Hormone Cautions

We also have the option of doing it unsafely, and that's the reason (probably the only valid reason) that you're likely to read about how dangerous hormones can be. That's true because hormone supplements are very different from the vitamins, minerals, and other supplements you may be taking. Although you can easily buy some hormone supplements at any health food store or pharmacy, these potent products, unlike most nutrients, have a very specific and narrow range of doses. They must be given in carefully measured doses, preferably under the supervision of an experienced physician. The goal is to achieve the ideal blood level of the hormone. Too little is inadequate. Too much can be dangerous in itself and quite likely to throw your other hormones out of synch. So, "doing it properly" means not only bringing the level of an undersupplied hormone up to an optimal level but also keeping it in balance with the other hormones.

At the Atkins Center, I use blood measurements to determine the hormone levels of my patients both before and after they start taking hormone supplements. The individual dosages are based on the starting measurements and then adjusted up or down as needed. To reap the best rewards from hormone optimization, you should find an experienced physician who can do the blood testing necessary to find the best dosages for you.

Mainstream endocrinologists are all keenly aware of the value of total hormonal balance, yet only a small minority of them actually take steps to help their patients achieve it. If you find yourself seeking the help of such a specialist, I suggest that you use this book as a guide to determine whether you are getting the best counseling.

The Hormone Philharmonic

Ideally, your hormones act in concert, just as an orchestra plays together in tune. When your hormones are all working properly with one another, your body is working at peak harmony—the physiological equivalent of an orchestra playing a symphony. But just as one instrument playing too vigorously can overpower the melodic line and throw the other musicians off, so too can too much of one hormone, whether produced in your body or taken as a supplement, overpower the other hormones and suppress their action.

That's the most important lesson of hormone therapy: You can totally deharmonize your endocrine balance by giving it too much of a single hormone. But, and this applies mainly to the steroid hormones (the group I'll be discussing the most), some hormones are more likely to cause this problem than others. To understand which are more likely to do this you must understand the process of differentiation your body uses to make hormones.

You make the steroid hormones through a complex process that begins with the much maligned yet essential chemical building block cholesterol. When your body determines that it needs cholesterol more to create steroid hormones than to make bile, nerve sheaths, or any of the various other cholesterol-based substances in your body, it converts the cholesterol into a rudimentary precursor chemical called a prohormone. Then, by the addition or deletion of a single molecule or a simple cluster of molecules, the prohormone is converted into a real hormone, such as cortisone or testosterone.

Generally, most hormonal biochemistry proceeds easily toward differentiating into the hormones your body perceives it needs. It's biochemically almost impossible to go in the other direction and return to an earlier stage of differentiation.

Let me present, as an example, the most common hormonal abnormality I see among my patients. It is almost unheard of to see a woman taking a full dose of hormone replacement therapy (with unnatural estrogens and progesterones) whose blood levels of DHEA, the hormone precursor I'll describe just below, are not considerably depleted. This happens because of a feedback loop in which an increased level of a differentiated hormone suppresses the manufacture of an earlier form of the hormone. It means she's likely to be deficient in a variety of important hormones derived from DHEA.

Let's learn about this in detail.

DHEA: The Mother Hormone

DHEA is often called the "mother" hormone because it's the precursor for the other adrenal hormones, including all the adrenal steroids, such as the stress hormone cortisol, and all the sex hormones, such as estrogen, progesterone, and testosterone. Of all the biomarkers for aging, DHEA (dehydroepiandrosterone) is perhaps the most telling. Study after study confirms that DHEA levels are an excellent predictor of age-related health problems.

The level of DHEA, in turn, is probably the most rapidly declining hormone as we age, starting in our midtwenties. The lower your DHEA, the more likely you are to have the degenerative diseases of accelerated aging: atherosclerosis, diabetes, cancer, osteoporosis, and lowered immunity. To put it more bluntly, the lower your DHEA, the more likely you are to die from an age-related disease.[1]

Conversely, high levels of DHEA may protect you from or even reverse precisely the same diseases. The higher your DHEA level, the better you feel, with a greater sense of overall well-being and a better ability to deal with emotional and physical stress.[2]

DHEA is the most abundant hormone in your body—ordinarily you make about 25 to 30 mg of it every day. If your DHEA production drops, so does your production of all the other related hormones.

Your adrenal glands manufacture DHEA from cholesterol (you also make very small amounts of DHEA in your testes or ovaries). Yes, that's the same cholesterol that consensus medicine insists is a dangerous substance that has no business being in your blood. Yet if your blood levels of cholesterol are inadequate, your body doesn't have the essential raw material to make the crucial hormone that's the precursor for more than forty other critical adrenal hormones. The cascade of hormone production is seriously disrupted, with predictably serious consequences for your health. Almost every patient I've given DHEA to, young or old, has shown dramatic improvement as soon as his or her DHEA level was restored to an optimal level.

Your levels of DHEA peak when you're between twenty and twenty-five. After that, the amount of DHEA you produce declines naturally at the rate of about 2 percent a year. That means that by the time you're forty or so, you're making only about half the DHEA you did at age twenty. At age sixty-five, you're down to only about 10 to 20 percent of your peak. At age eighty, you're making only about 5 percent of your peak. In general, women make about 10 to 20 percent less DHEA than men; their rate of production still declines at the same 2 percent a year.

DHEA and Heart Disease

Low DHEA is a much better predictor than high cholesterol of heart attack, yet your doctor is very unlikely to test your DHEA level.[3] In fact, your doctor will probably treat your high cholesterol with a statin drug that works by preventing the manufacture of cholesterol and thereby further reduces your production of DHEA. Exactly the opposite approach is far better. Taking DHEA supplements will also lower your LDL cholesterol, but without the side effects of statin drugs. At the same time, the DHEA will lower your chances of having a dangerous blood clot. Of course, you'll also be enjoying all the other benefits of increased DHEA levels.[4]

There's a definite correlation between DHEA levels and coronary artery disease. To give just one example, a particularly interesting study of patients about to have coronary bypass operations showed that the higher their DHEA, the less severe was their coronary artery disease.[5]

Enhancing Immunity with DHEA

A twenty-year-old can quickly shake off a cold or flu that would keep a sixty-year-old sick for a week. As you age, your immune system gets weaker, making you more susceptible to illness and infection. Your aging immune system also makes you more susceptible to degenerative diseases such as atherosclerosis and autoimmune diseases. If you could restore your immune system to its youthful level, wouldn't you? You can, with DHEA. This amazing hormone has been shown to increase the production of antibodies and increase the activity of infection-fighting immune cells such as monocytes and natural killer cells.

In 1997, a careful study of healthy older men showed just how well DHEA enhances immunity. The test subjects took 50 mg of DHEA a day for twenty weeks. At the end of that time, all the men showed remarkable increases in immune components in their blood. Most notably, their levels of white blood cells, called monocytes, increased on average by 45 percent; other markers such as T cells went up by at least 20 percent.[6]

I see the evidence for the immune-enhancing function of DHEA every day in my patients. At the Atkins Center we prescribe it for all patients with impaired immunity. It's particularly effective for patients with chronic fatigue syndrome or with autoimmune ailments such as rheumatoid arthritis and lupus. Virtually all of these patients have surprisingly low levels of DHEA; after they have been on DHEA for just a few weeks, I see a strong improvement in their overall immune function. The patients feel much better; symptoms such as depression and fatigue are usually much improved.

Cancer and DHEA

It's not a cure, but DHEA could be something even better: a supplement that prevents cancer from occurring. Animal studies show that DHEA prevents cancers of the breast, colon, liver, lungs, prostate, lymphatic system, and skin. I first learned about using DHEA for any medical purpose in the 1970s, when alternative oncologists in Germany began using it successfully with their cancer patients.

Your chances of getting cancer rise as your DHEA levels fall—people with bladder cancer and women with breast cancer almost always have much lower than normal DHEA levels.[7] All the evidence points toward a strong role for DHEA as a cancer preventive, even if the definitive studies have yet to be done.

One known exception: A man at risk for prostate cancer, or one who already has it, needs to be very cautious about using DHEA. I believe he can still benefit from this helpful hormone, but he needs to be monitored carefully by a physician. DHEA can increase testosterone production, which in turn could feed prostate cancer. To use DHEA safely, he needs to have frequent PSA blood tests to monitor his risk of prostate cancer. A useful alternative here is 7-keto DHEA, a variation that leads to the development of the adrenal hormones but not testosterone (or other sex hormones) production.

Stronger Bones with DHEA

DHEA not only can stop osteoporosis, it can reverse it. This is how it works: DHEA increases the activity of bone-building cells called osteoblasts and inhibits the activity of bone-destroying cells called osteoclasts.

People with osteoporosis generally have much lower levels of DHEA than people who don't. Similarly, among older adults, the people with the highest DHEA levels have the densest bones. We know from animal studies that DHEA supplements can actually restore lost bone density.[8] Can it do the same for you? I think it can, which is why I use DHEA supplements to

create optimal blood levels for all my patients—male and female—who are at risk for osteoporosis.

Taking DHEA

All the above strongly suggests that you should be aware of
your DHEA level and supplement it if it's low. I have found no
problems when trying to restore the blood levels of my patients
to what is optimal for a thirty-year-old; in older patients, the
goal is to achieve the level of someone in his or her twenties or
thirties. For women, that's ideally between 200 and 300 units;
for men, between 300 and 400.

The Cortisol Connection

The prohormones, defined as those capable of developing into
a variety of differentiated hormones, are very unlikely to lead
to a hormonal imbalance, because the body has so many different options of what it can convert these precursors to. The body
itself determines which derivatives it needs most. Further,
DHEA and its companion prohormones are among the few
hormones in your body that don't have a feedback mechanism
for turning off other hormones when you take supplements.
When your body has too much or too little of most other hormones, feedback mechanisms signal your glands to speed up
or slow down their production. But so far as we know, your
body doesn't respond to DHEA supplements by shutting down
its own production.

   Your normal DHEA production is counteracted, in a very
complex process, by the adrenal hormone cortisol. Sometimes

called the stress hormone, cortisol is made in your adrenal glands and secreted when your body needs it. It's the second most abundant hormone in your body after DHEA—you usually make about 10 to 20 mg a day. When you're under stress, however, you make a lot more cortisol, and that in turn inhibits your production of DHEA. As time goes by and you age, the combination of naturally decreasing DHEA production plus the continual stress many of us are under from work and family pressures causes a relative increase in cortisol, which can lead to a serious hormonal imbalance. Your DHEA production, already naturally lower, gets further suppressed by excess cortisol. Your hormonal harmony gets out of balance as the cortisol gradually takes over. Instead of symphony, you have a cacophony.

Too much cortisol and not enough DHEA has major ramifications for your health. As the cortisol pushes out the DHEA, all your other hormones are affected as well. In particular, the cortisol-DHEA connection is closely related to the insulin-glucagon connection. As your cortisol level rises, so does your insulin level. Once you start getting excess cortisol in your system, the aging process accelerates. Not only do you lose the protection of DHEA, the cortisol also inhibits your production of eicosanoids, the short-lived chemical messengers that carry out the order sent by your hormones.

Clearly, restoring the balance between your DHEA and cortisol levels is crucial to breaking this deadly aging cycle. One major step in that direction is to reduce your cortisol level, so that your body will be able to make and use as much of your natural DHEA as possible. Because cortisol is the stress hormone, one good way to lower your levels of it is to lower your stress levels. The more reliable way may be to use some of the vitanutrients that work well to bring those levels down, such as acetyl-l-carnitine, vitamin C, vitamin A, zinc, and selenium.

DHEA Doses

The other part of the DHEA-cortisol reduction equation is DHEA supplements. As a starting dose, I generally prescribe 10 to 30 mg of DHEA to women and 30 to 50 mg to men. I then adjust the dose over the next few months until the desired blood level is reached. DHEA has very few side effects, but at high doses there may be unwanted hair growth in women, acne, irritability, and insomnia. In some very rare cases, people taking high doses may develop heart palpitations or irregular heartbeats.

Although DHEA is the precursor hormone to estrogen, in practice it doesn't seem to raise estrogen levels much if at all. Almost all of a woman's estrogen is produced in her ovaries. Based on the current research, it's unlikely that taking DHEA supplements will raise your risk of breast cancer. In fact, DHEA has long been part of the breast cancer *treatment* protocols of several European alternative cancer therapists.

Today many reputable manufacturers produce pharmaceutical-grade DHEA. To make DHEA, a sterol called diosgenin is extracted from wild yams. Diosgenin needs to be manipulated through at least six steps in the laboratory to convert it into DHEA. You may encounter products that claim to be "wild yam extract," "DHEA precursor," or "natural DHEA." Since your body can't begin to transform wild yam extract into DHEA, these products are not what you're looking for. There is no reason to consider any product that doesn't clearly state the dose of DHEA in milligrams on the label.

Pregnenolone: The Grandmother Hormone

If DHEA can be called the mother hormone, then pregnenolone is the "grandmother" hormone. Cholesterol in your body is converted to pregnenolone as the first biochemical step in making all your other steroid hormones. Pregnenolone is, in fact, the direct precursor of DHEA, which the body then converts into a range of other hormones, such as androstenedione and androstenediol, which are then converted into the hormones testosterone, estradiol and its derivatives, cortisol, and aldosterone.

Pregnenolone's main advantage is that it is also converted into progesterone. Because that conversion takes place one step before pregnenolone is converted into DHEA, the grandmother hormone can be vital for women by creating a balance with estrogen. (I'll come back to this point for more discussion in the next chapter.)

Your pregnenolone production peaks when you're in your early thirties, then steadily declines. By the time you reach your seventies, your pregnenolone production is down to just about 40 percent of your peak.[9] A decline in pregnenolone production is a natural part of growing older, but you can accelerate the decline by starving your body of cholesterol. An overly strict, cholesterol-free vegetarian diet could deprive you of the essential raw materials from which pregnenolone is made. Another pathway to this deprivation is provided by the statin family of cholesterol-lowering drugs. If either, or both, apply to you, you have a formula for unnaturally reduced pregnenolone production. And since pregnenolone is the grandmother hormone, making less of it for whatever reason means you also make less of all the other hormones down the line, with all the predictable negative consequences.

Pregnenolone was discovered back in the 1940s. Researchers were interested in it once they found that adrenal hormones could suppress the pain and swelling of rheumatoid arthritis. They found that pregnenolone was the only hormone that helped relieve the symptoms without the metabolic side effects the other hormones induced. Despite this, they turned their attention to hydrocortisone and its derivatives. This is the origin of the corticosteroid drugs such as prednisone that were originally hailed as "miracle drugs." Today these drugs are seen for what they are: dangerous artificial substances that cause such a wide range of adverse side effects that they cannot be taken in high doses for more than a brief period.

At the Atkins Center we use natural pregnenolone supplements (generally along with DHEA) to treat problems that conventional physicians treat with prednisone. Pregnenolone isn't quite as powerful or fast acting, but it is much less likely to cause elevated blood pressure, weight gain, diabetes, or fluid retention. We find it to be very helpful for treating arthritis and autoimmune diseases such as lupus and multiple sclerosis. Since we feel that pregnenolone and DHEA should be in balance, we use comparable amounts of each.

Pregnenolone is the precursor hormone for the female hormone progesterone. In fact, some of a woman's pregnenolone is converted directly to progesterone without any intermediate steps. Because pregnenolone is a very safe hormone that doesn't really have any metabolic side effects (although high doses can cause mild water retention), it is high on my list of natural substances that help balance a woman's hormone-related health problems.

One reason your DHEA production drops as you age is that your pregnenolone production also drops, as does your production of the enzyme that converts pregnenolone to DHEA. Taking pregnenolone supplements, which are now available over the counter, may not increase your DHEA level. Taking pregnenolone and DHEA supplements together, however, could do a lot to restore optimal levels of both hormones. This may have the advantage of also turning down your production of cortisol.

To help restore youthful levels of pregnenolone in my patients, I usually start with doses of 20 to 40 mg daily. If, after a few months, the level hasn't gone up enough, I might raise the dose. How you will react to pregnenolone is unpredictable. Don't try taking supplements on your own—you need to work with an experienced physician who can use blood tests at regular intervals to monitor your levels and optimize your dosage.

As I'm sure you appreciate by now, hormone optimization is a complex subject. Raising your levels of the hormones I've just discussed will certainly help you regain some of your youthful vigor and health, but they're just the first step. In the next chapter I'll explain how you can improve your levels of hormones that may truly be able to turn back the clock.

13

Hormones That Turn Back the Clock

Can any single hormone truly turn back the clock on aging? Can any one vitanutrient bring you back to the youthful health and vigor you enjoyed in your twenties and thirties? No. There are no magic bullets against aging. But the entire premise of this book is that *in combination* the right vitanutrients, along with the right diet and lifestyle, can certainly slow down the clock and perhaps stop it or even turn it back. In this chapter you'll learn about the vitanutrients that are most effective for restoring low levels of steroid hormones such as testosterone and progesterone. You'll also learn about natural, safe ways to eliminate menopause symptoms and lower your risk of osteoporosis. And you'll learn about one of the most exciting and controversial new developments in hormone optimization: human growth hormone.

Androstenedione and Natural Testosterone

Even if you're not a sports fan like me, you must have heard about Mark McGwire's record-smashing seventy home runs in the 1998 season. A bit of controversy went along with the record, because McGwire openly acknowledged his use of an over-the-counter hormone supplement called androstenedione. Let me point out that although using androstenedione is perfectly legal in major league baseball, it is banned by many other sports organizations. The reason? The sports officials say androstenedione is an anabolic steroid—that is, a steroid hormone that builds muscle. The officials are more than a little off base here. Androstenedione is indeed a steroid, but that's a very different animal from the artificial anabolic steroid drugs that are rightly banned in all sports. Artificial anabolic steroids such as methyltestosterone, like all artificial hormones, are unnatural substances that your body is not at all equipped to deal with. Instead of being cleared from your system naturally and easily through your normal metabolic pathways, as androstenedione and other natural hormones are, these drugs break down into toxic by-products that can do serious harm to your liver and may even cause cancer.

Since most of us aren't professional athletes, and since androstenedione is sold legally at pharmacies and health food stores, and since it is safe to use in reasonable doses, there's no reason not to take it—if it's right for you.

But when is it right for you? That's a good question. Generally speaking, androstenedione is said to produce a brief rise in your testosterone level that lasts for only a few hours. It's not all that clear from the few studies that have been done if androstenedione raises your testosterone level enough to have any real impact. But my experience using androstenedione in combination with DHEA indicates that a significant level of testosterone can be achieved, and, in fact, serum testosterone levels can be used to monitor androstenedione dosage.

I usually recommend androstenedione to my patients when I feel they will benefit from testosterone, and I usually give it with DHEA. The dosage is whatever produces optimal levels of DHEA and testosterone. Let me tell you why I like to optimize the testosterone level.

Testosterone Tales

Some of my male patients first come to me seeking help for vague problems such as fatigue, loss of muscle strength, insomnia, and depression. Others have more specific problems, such as heart disease or osteoporosis. And some are having the very specific problem of erectile difficulty or loss of sexual desire. What they often all have in common is very low testosterone levels. They're producing only a fraction of the free testosterone they need to remain active, vital, and healthy. Testosterone levels, like most of the steroid hormones I've been discussing, drop with advancing years. I like to see to it that my older patients achieve levels normal for a man in his thirties.

To a degree, making less testosterone as you age is perfectly normal. Men naturally begin to make less testosterone as they enter their fifties, just as women naturally begin to produce less of the female hormones. In fact, the process in men is in many ways so similar to that in women that it's often called male menopause or andropause.

Like menopausal women, andropausal men in their late forties and early fifties experience increases in body fat, a greater risk of cardiovascular disease and osteoporosis, depression, and forgetfulness. The major difference is that a woman can use a monthly marker—her menstrual period—to be aware of the changes in her body. Men don't have a similar marker. Even if they did, many would ignore it. What man likes to think that the hormone that defines his very maleness could possibly be diminishing in his body?

The truth is, men, that our testosterone production does slowly decline as we age, generally for one or more reasons. The most common cause is a natural decrease in the number of testosterone-producing Leydig cells in your testes as you age. The fewer Leydig cells you have, the less testosterone you make. Another common cause of decreased testosterone is an increase in SHBG, the protein that binds sex hormones and makes it unavailable to your body. For reasons we don't really understand yet, you make more SHBG as you age.

Other factors can reduce the activity of your Leydig cells. An excess of the female hormone estradiol suppresses the function of the Leydig cells. All men produce some estradiol as a normal function of producing testosterone, but ordinarily you have a good balance between lots of testosterone and a little estradiol. As you age, though, the balance can get thrown off.

One good way to get your testosterone/estradiol balance out of whack is to have a major spare tire around your middle. In a complicated metabolic process, the excess fat makes your testosterone level drop and your estradiol level rise, with very undesirable effects on your sexuality and health.

Of course, losing that spare tire means losing weight, a project that is laughably easy to those who know my low-carbohydrate diet, as you will do once you've made a commitment to follow the program I outline in *Dr. Atkins' New Diet Revolution*.

Sometimes low testosterone is caused by following the standard medical advice to eat a low-fat diet. I find this to be particularly true for my patients with cardiovascular disease. Their fear of the dreaded dietary cholesterol leads them to go on low-fat diets, with the hearty approval of their conventional cardiologists. They starve their bodies of the cholesterol they need to make testosterone. The paradox of these misguided efforts is that testosterone has a protective effect on the heart and actually improves blood lipid profiles.[1]

Other supplements short of testosterone supplements may also help. Supplemental DHEA, which is easily converted into testosterone, is often very valuable. And I am convinced that androstenedione brings out DHEA's effect of raising testosterone. Equally critical are the anticortisol nutrients I listed back in Chapter 12. When your cortisol levels are high, your DHEA levels are low; your testosterone level is also low because you don't have enough of the precursor. Counteract the cortisol and your DHEA level, and thus your testosterone level, will rise.

There still remain men for whom all these measures fail to raise their testosterone levels back up to our goal levels. For these cases I prescribe supplements of natural testosterone. I emphasize the natural part of that prescription. Over the years, pharmaceutical companies have patented a wide variety of unnatural testosterone supplements, otherwise known as anabolic steroid drugs.

Recently some drug manufacturers have discovered that although they can't patent natural testosterone, they can still profit from it by providing easy and painless ways to administer it. Today natural testosterone is available in skin patches, skin creams and gels, and a sublingual (under the tongue) tablet. These new delivery systems make it easy for patients to give themselves a steady, exact dose on a daily basis. Since testosterone is a controlled substance requiring a triplicate prescription, you need to work with your doctor to determine the right dosage for you.

Natural testosterone is a very effective treatment, but all testosterone products need to be used with caution. In particular, men who have a history of prostate cancer should not use it—although there's no evidence to show that taking testosterone will cause prostate cancer. To be on the safe side, I always screen patients for prostate cancer using the prostate-specific antigen (PSA) blood test.

One word of warning: Taking testosterone can cause a transient rise in your PSA level. If you're planning to have a routine PSA blood test, don't use testosterone for a few days before.

Testosterone for Women

All women naturally produce small amounts of testosterone. Just as a woman's production of female hormones declines with age, so too does her production of testosterone. It's the major reason that many menopausal women report declining libido and less satisfaction from sex—even those already using female hormone replacement therapy. Because the dose needed to restore a woman's normal testosterone level is quite small, I don't like to prescribe it—it's too easy to give an unnecessarily large amount. Instead, I prefer to use DHEA and/or androstenedione, which are converted naturally into testosterone in the body. When I see a small but measurable rise in testosterone, and along with it, a noticeable improvement in sexual desire, then we've achieved our goal.

Progesterone: Menopause the Natural Way

There may not be a more controversial area of hormone optimization than hormone replacement therapy (HRT) in menopause. Standard medical treatment calls for women who have stopped menstruating to be given a combination of estrogen and progesterone. These artificial hormones, which differ substantially from the hormones they are said to replace, are heavily advertised in medical journals and enthusiastically endorsed by the medical establishment. Prescribing HRT for women over fifty has become almost automatic for many physicians.

The only problem is that the combination of estrogen and progesterone can be, for a woman already hormonally imbalanced, downright dangerous to her health. The combination will make most women with a weight-gaining tendency gain weight, even if they are a normal weight when they start. It will certainly keep women from losing weight if they are overweight. If you already have an insulin-related disorder such as low blood sugar, diabetes, high triglycerides, or high blood pressure, HRT will make the problems worse. If you're on the borderline for an insulin-related disorder, HRT could tip you over into a full-blown version of it.

Whenever I wear my other hat, that of a weight-control guru with a diet able to provide weight loss in more than 99 percent of those who follow it, I note the true magnitude of the HRT problem. It inhibits weight loss, even to the point of turning my weight-loss diet into a weight-gaining experience. In case you're wondering how often that happens, I can report that I've seen it in more than three thousand patients.

Here's why. Progesterone has been a known weight-gaining hormone since 1976. That's when the famed Swedish metabolic researcher Per Bjorntorp described animal studies showing an increase in the size of fat cells along with a sevenfold increase in plasma insulin levels.[2]

Meanwhile, the estrogen component of HRT inhibits the one hormone that tries to neutralize the effects of insulin—glucagon. Giving estradiol to women cuts down glucagon secretion and allows the blood lipids to elevate.[3]

With so much basic research indicating that HRT has adverse effects on glucose/insulin metabolism, it's amazing how few doctors who prescribe it are aware of the problems they are causing.

Do the supposed benefits of HRT balance out the disadvantages? I don't think so. The mantra conventional doctors repeat over and over is that HRT prevents cardiovascular disease. The mantra is based on numerous epidemiologic studies showing that women who take hormones do considerably better. But a recent study, done more scientifically and involving twenty medical centers nationwide, has shown that a new mantra is badly needed. Nearly three thousand women participated in the four-year Heart and Estrogen/Progestin Replacement Study (HERS), with half taking a hormone replacement formula and half taking a placebo. The researchers were dismayed to find that over the four years, fifty-eight of the placebo-group women died of heart attacks, while seventy-one of the HRT-group women died of heart attacks. In other words, the HRT group had a 23 percent increase in heart attack deaths.[4] Why? One reason may be that the HRT raised their triglyceride levels past the danger point and into the fatal range.

Despite the disappointing results of HERS, most conventional doctors point to the dozens of other studies that showed that HRT lowers cardiovascular disease rates. What they conveniently overlook is that all of these studies have a fundamental flaw—they are retrospective. Identical groups were not selected for comparison, and that's a scientific no-no. What the studies analyzed were women taking HRT because of their own decision and/or that of their doctors. The control groups were women who decided by themselves not to be on HRT. Menopausal women who aren't in particularly good health—they're overweight, or they have diabetes, asthma, or high blood pressure, for instance—often don't use HRT, because they find it makes their problems worse. The women who seek out and continue to use HRT tend to be healthier, slimmer, and more dedicated to lifestyle improvements. In other words, they're less likely to have heart disease with or without HRT.

In fairness, let me say that the standard estrogen/progesterone combination used in HRT does indeed lower your total cholesterol and does raise your level of good HDL cholesterol. On the other hand, as mentioned, HRT can sharply elevate that other serious risk factor for heart disease, your triglyceride level. The upward jump could be 30 percent or more.

There is a much better, much more natural way to use hormones to treat the unpleasant effects of menopause, such as mood swings, hot flashes, vaginal dryness, and so on—natural progesterone. Combined with the right vitanutrients, natural progesterone gives real protection not only against menopausal symptoms but also against the other scourges of older women, osteoporosis and heart disease.

The approach I use at the Atkins Center is a natural progesterone skin cream, combined with the use of vitanutrient supplements. The cream is very easy to use—simply rub about a teaspoon into the skin every night at bedtime for twenty-one days; often I recommend taking a week off and then starting again. Natural progesterone creams are available over the counter at pharmacies and health food stores. Various products have different amounts of natural progesterone. Be sure you know how much you're getting. The best products contain 3 percent natural progesterone.

The most important of the vitanutrients in treating menopause symptoms is folic acid in prescription-strength doses of 30 to 60 mg. Doses this large stimulate natural estrogen production in women and also have an estrogenlike effect that helps to minimize many of the symptoms of menopause. They also consistently stimulate a woman's libido.

The second menopause-correcting vitanutrient is the mineral boron. This trace mineral has been found to increase estrogen and progesterone levels and to be an effective therapy for osteoporosis, possibly independent of its effect on hormones. I prescribe between 10 and 20 mg daily of boron; women generally notice an improvement within a few weeks.

Add to this the most estrogenic of foods, the soybean and its derivatives, and herbs such as black cohosh and others, and you can readily see that there are many elements to choose from to create a successful alternative to HRT.

Most of my patients who take this route find that it relieves their menopause symptoms so well that they avoid hormone replacement therapy altogether. Almost all of the rest find that they can at least lower their doses of synthetic hormones. And this becomes our endpoint. I prefer to have a woman take the smallest amount of estrogen that still controls her menopause symptoms. That way, the adverse effect of estrogenic hormones on raising insulin levels is kept to a minimum.

Building Bones with Progesterone

When HRT enthusiasts learn that the cardiovascular disease mantra is not supportable, they fall back to reciting the osteoporosis mantra. It is true that HRT slows down osteoporosis a bit, but it does very little to prevent or reverse it. In fact, estrogen loss has less of an effect on bone loss than you have been led to believe. Osteoporosis begins in your late thirties, when your estrogen levels are still normal. By the time you reach your fifties and menopause, you've been slowly losing bone mass for some twenty years.

After menopause, bone loss accelerates, sometimes to the point of crippling fractures from even the simplest exertion. But it's less the lack of estrogen that causes osteoporosis than the lack of progesterone.

We know from studies that estrogen replacement therapy can slow the breakdown of bone—but only if it's taken during the three to five years around the onset of menopause. After that, estrogen doesn't do much if anything to slow bone loss.

Natural progesterone (the term defines the prohormone rather than the synthetic analogs that are most frequently prescribed) can actually build new bone, enough to balance out or even overcome bone loss. In short, progesterone supplements can help reverse osteoporosis by stimulating the growth of solid new bone.[5]

The vast majority of Atkins Center patients with decreased bone density have had good results with the natural approach to reversing—not just slowing—osteoporosis. It's safe, relatively inexpensive—and it works. The first step is using natural progesterone, folic acid, and boron in the amounts described earlier. A newly available supplement called ipriflavone (IP), made from isoflavones (natural plant estrogens), improves bone density just as estrogen does, but without the potential dangers. In fact, just the opposite happens. Estrogen can increase your risk of cancer, while ipriflavone can reduce it.[6]

I recommend taking 600 mg of ipriflavone daily, in doses spread out over the day. In addition, you'll need to take supplements of some important vitanutrients such as vitamin D, calcium, magnesium, and strontium, as well as vitamin K. Finally, weight-bearing exercise helps keep your bones strong. Taking a brisk walk for twenty minutes three times a week or doing aerobics is a good start in the right direction.

Thinking About Thyroid

Because I practice complementary medicine, it's amazing how few drug prescriptions I write. Of the ones I do, though, nearly half are for thyroid hormone. Like the other hormones I've discussed, your production of thyroid hormone naturally diminishes somewhat with age. Low thyroid production is a subtle and often undiagnosed cause of aging. It increases your risk of heart disease, and the mental confusion it causes can sometimes be mistaken for senility.

Even though easily 25 percent of the adult population suffers from mild to severe hypothyroidism (low thyroid function), the problem is frequently left undiagnosed. (The opposite problem, an overactive thyroid, *hyper*thyroidism is relatively rare.) That's because most conventional doctors diagnose it by relying only on blood tests of your levels of the thyroid hormones T4 (also called thyroxine), T3 (your body converts T4 to T3), and another hormone called TSH (thyroid stimulating hormone, which is produced by your pituitary gland). The normal range for all three of these hormones is extremely broad, however. Your results could be half the average level and still be considered within normal limits.

That is exactly the reason you need a nonlaboratory clinical evaluation whenever an underactive thyroid is even faintly suspected. Your blood test might show that your thyroid function is within those very broad normal limits, but you may still be having the symptoms of hypothyroidism, including sensitivity to cold, weight gain or inability to lose weight, fatigue and lethargy, depression, dry skin, and elevated cholesterol levels. For the latter reason, low thyroid function may be an under-recognized cause of atherosclerosis.

Let's look more closely at what your thyroid does and why it might start to fail.

One of your thyroid gland's major functions is to regulate your body temperature, which is why sensitivity to cold is one of the earliest symptoms of hypothyroidism. Your thyroid's other main function is to regulate the speed of your metabolism. When your thyroid is underactive, your metabolism slows, which is why the other early symptoms of hypothyroidism are tiredness and weight gain.

What makes your thyroid stop functioning well? Occasionally, the problem is nutritional. You need the amino acid tyrosine and the mineral iodine to make T4, and you need the minerals zinc and selenium to produce the enzyme that converts T4 to T3.

Nutritional deficiency is only rarely the cause of hypothyroidism, however. Often the cause is autoimmune thyroiditis (also known as Hashimoto's disease), in which your own antibodies attack your thyroid. We don't really know why this happens, but I believe that many cases can be traced to root canal work done to keep a dead tooth in your mouth.

Another major cause of hypothyroidism is your body's own efforts to preserve its status quo (technically, to achieve homeostasis). Hypothyroidism is an extremely common result of being on a weight-loss diet, my kind or anyone else's, for any real length of time. Your body resists losing weight and thus alters its homeostasis by reducing its production of thyroid hormone.

No matter what the cause, the answer to the problem is the same—take the hormone in question. I recommend taking a natural (animal) thyroid supplement over the synthetic kind, particularly when hypothyroidism is caused by advancing age or dieting. I prescribe the synthetic hormone only in cases of autoimmune disease, where your own immune system might destroy the natural hormone.

The Therapeutic Trial

The problem with supplementing the thyroid is that more often than not there is a discrepancy between what the lab tests show and what the clinical picture shows. Your lab results might well be in the normal range, but you might be having the symptoms of hypothyroidism, particularly if your body temperature is consistently low (97.8° F or even lower). You and your doctor may legitimately be wondering if you really need supplemental thyroid.

Whenever the question is validly raised, my answer is to try it and see if you benefit—in other words, do a therapeutic trial. It's important to remember that such a trial is not without risk, because an overdose of thyroid hormone (or natural over-production) creates hyperthyroidism, with symptoms such as rapid heartbeat, heart palpitations or rhythm problems, nervousness, jitteriness, sweating, and insomnia.

Even so, a therapeutic trial is quite safe as long as you start with an extremely low dose and slowly increase it while carefully tracking your body temperature, pulse rate, and the progress of any other symptoms. Most patients with hypothyroidism end up with a dose of 1 to 3 g, but the dose is not as important as the way you and your doctor decide you're taking the right amount. The goal is to achieve the maximum feeling of well-being while making sure the pulse is still normal (below 80 beats per minute), raising the body temperature closer to normal, relieving the fatigue, dry skin, and other symptoms, and creating no new symptoms. Once you've found the appropriate dose, you still need to see your doctor at regular intervals to make sure the situation hasn't changed and that the dose is still the right one for you.

Human Growth Hormone: Real Rejuvenation—with Your Doctor's Help

If you decide to check out the growing number of antiaging clinics that are springing up all over the United States, you will quickly discover that the treatment at many of them is based on the almost routine prescribing and administering of human growth hormone (HGH) and/or substances related to it.

There are two reasons for this phenomenon. One: Patients expect to pay at least $12,000 a year for such treatment, and somewhere in that amount is the possibility of significant profit to the clinic. Two: There can be, and usually is, a very impressive group of beneficial responses to HGH.

These two facts have led to a thriving business opportunity for entrepreneurial doctors, but they carry with them a risk that cannot go unnoticed. I feel that a tendency arises to administer HGH to people who may not need it. This is very undesirable, because these people could actually be harmed by a hormonal imbalance created by the treatment. The counterweight to this is that giving HGH requires a doctor's care—it is clearly not a do-it-yourself proposition. No reputable clinic would administer HGH without careful blood tests to monitor levels of the hormone.

Having said all that, let me now say that I believe HGH is one of the most intriguing new hormone-optimizing substances available today. As I explain to you what all the excitement is about, I will have to get a little technical. Please follow along—you'll need this information to understand the tremendous potential of human growth hormone.

As its name suggests, human growth hormone tells your body to grow and to maintain and repair itself. The word "anabolic," which means "building up tissues and functions," applies perfectly to HGH. In addition, HGH is extremely important for your metabolism—it's involved with just about every aspect of helping your body use energy and remove wastes. It also tells your body when to release fat from body tissues to be burned for energy.

Your endocrine system is a very complex, delicately balanced arrangement of feedback loops, all designed to keep your body running normally on an even keel. HGH is, quantitatively, the major hormone put out by your pituitary gland, which is found at the base of your brain. When the pituitary gland gets a message from the other gland-stimulating part of your brain, the hypothalamus, it releases HGH. The HGH then gets carried to your liver, where it stimulates the production of hormone-like substances known as insulin growth factors. The most pertinent of these is insulin growth factor 1 (IGF-1), since it works directly with HGH to regulate your metabolism and promote growth. Indeed, IGF-1 can be administered along with HGH, or separately, to achieve nearly identical results.

HGH is released by your pituitary in a cycle of short bursts throughout the day, roughly once every four hours or so. About 70 percent of your HGH production comes at night while you are in deep sleep. (Your level of IGF-1, however, remains fairly constant throughout the day.)

Once enough HGH has been released, the hypothalamus sends a second message to your pituitary, using a hormone called somatostatin (also known as GH inhibiting factor). Somatostatin tells your pituitary gland to stop making HGH for the moment. Your production of somatostatin seems to increase with age. That may be one reason your HGH level, which reaches its peak during your teens, gradually drops off at the rate of about 14 percent per decade. By the time you're age sixty or so, you're making only abut 25 percent of the HGH you made when you were twenty.

Growth Hormone Deficiency Syndrome

If your HGH drops a little too far or fast, you can classified as being deficient in growth hormone. In 1990, Dr. Dan Rudman, who was one of my instructors during my residency at the

Goldwater Hospital division of Columbia University, told the world about the exciting benefits of HGH. Dr. Rudman has defined the criterion for diagnosing growth hormone deficiency as an IGF-1 level below 350 IU. Some 30 percent of apparently healthy sixty-year-old men are below this level. That statistic provides a good guesstimate of how many people should be trying in some way to optimize their IGF-1 level.

Hundreds of scientific studies have been published describing recent findings in growth hormone deficiency (GHD).[7] The studies show that the symptoms of GHD include an increase in body fat with a simultaneous decrease in lean body mass, muscle bulk, and muscle strength. Bone density is decreased in GHD, and fractures from osteoporosis occur more often. Kidney and lung function impairment have been reported as well.

Perhaps the organ most vulnerable to low levels of growth hormone is the heart. People with growth hormone deficiency have also been found to have elevated risk factors for heart disease: high triglycerides, low HDL, and elevated LDL. This suggests that insulin resistance, one of the major problems identified in this book, would be found quite often among people with GHD—and, in fact, it is.[8]

HGH and Obesity

Growth hormone deficiency is made considerably worse if you are overweight, because obesity lowers your level of human growth hormone every bit as much as advancing age does. The heavier you are, the less HGH you will have; the less body fat you have, the more HGH you will have.[9]

HGH as Treatment

You have every right to assume that all of the aforementioned manifestations of growth hormone deficiency can be corrected, at least in part, by administering HGH. But HGH may do much more! Although the idea of using HGH to fight some of the conditions of aging may date back to the work in the 1960s of another one of my mentors, Dr. Vladimir Dilman, the floodgates of research were opened by the breakthrough study headed by Dr. Daniel Rudman and published in the *New England Journal of Medicine* in 1990. Dr. Rudman studied healthy, albeit frail and elderly, men whose IGF-1 levels were below 350 units. He treated twelve of them with a three-times-a-week injected dose of HGH. The study's conclusion, that "the effects of six months of HGH on the lean body mass and adipose tissue mass of the men were equivalent in magnitude to the changes incurred during ten to twenty years of aging," set off the HGH revolution.[10]

Among the impressive studies are that HGH (or IGF-1, or both) has helped in the treatment of a variety of heart disorders such as congestive heart failure and cardiomyopathy.[11] That means I look at the IGF-1 levels of all my heart patients who also have a decreased ability to exert themselves at a normal pace. Part of the treatment plan is to raise low IGF-1 levels back up to normal.

IGF-1 and Victory over Diabetes

To me, the area of clinical study that most closely ties HGH into my premise of what causes aging is the work on diabetes. Most of this research has been done using HGH's kissing cousin, IGF-1. Quite a few studies confirm that, rather than mimicking the action of insulin, as the name "insulinlike growth factor" suggests, IGF-1 works to combat insulin *resistance*. That means it lowers both the blood sugar *and* the insulin levels, thus avoiding the need to grasp either horn of the glucose/insulin dilemma. I am particularly excited by a joint study out of the Harvard and North Carolina medical complexes in which both blood sugar and insulin resistance were lowered dramatically.[12] The study was published in the journal *Diabetes*, which is standard reading for all doctors concerned with this disease. All diabetologists should have read it, but just try to find one who will give you HGH or IGF-1.

In addition, HGH has been used successfully to treat fibromyalgia,[13] to overcome wasting in HIV/AIDS and other conditions,[14] and as an effective treatment for obesity.[15]

The Downside

HGH and IGF-1, although they are natural substances, are prescription drugs, as well they should be. They have real, worrisome side effects: water retention, to the point of worsening heart failure even while strengthening the heart; joint pain, including temporomandibular joint problems and carpal tunnel syndrome; increases in heart rate and blood pressure; shortness of breath; headache; and fatigue.

Both my practice experience and my reading of the medical journals convince me that most of these problems are dose-related. They've been reported because of the practice in the research studies of giving a standard dose without frequently checking before-and-after blood levels and lowering the dose as needed. By modifying the protocols to use smaller doses and to accept more modest elevations of IGF-1 levels as evidence of improvement, we can avoid virtually all side effects.

How to Raise Your IGF-1

We've come a long way from Dr. Rudman's three-doses-a-week protocol. We have since learned that by synchronizing the administration of the HGH dose with the body's natural release of HGH at night we can raise the IGF-1 levels with a considerably smaller dose, which means considerably less cost. Because your body puts out HGH in brief pulsations, and because most of these occur soon after you fall asleep, I recommend taking a small dose every night at bedtime. A preferable method, suitable for those of you who regularly awaken during the night, is to take a half dose at bedtime and the second half with the first awakening.

This technique, along with starting with a low dose, allows the total dosage to be reduced without sacrificing effectiveness. I usually start my patients with a dosage of 0.0125 units per kilogram of weight per day. (A 220-pound person weighs 100 kg and would therefore start with a nightly dose of 1.25 units. A 176-pound person weighs 80 kg and would therefore take 1 unit daily.) I start patients on HGH in exactly the same way as I start them on any other hormone that can involve considerable risk, such as thyroid. I begin with an amount low enough to avoid any dose-related problems, check to see what that accomplishes both with regard to blood levels of IGF-1 and to clinical results and symptom control, and gradually work up the dosage scale until the desired improvement is achieved.

I am inclined to treat people with IGF-1 levels below 350 (400 in a younger person) with the goal of bringing it up to 600 (higher in a younger person). I have found, however, that if I can get *all* of the other hormones—DHEA, pregnenolone, androstenedione, testosterone, estrogen, progesterone, and thyroid—into an optimal range, then it's seldom necessary to bring the IGF-1 to a high level.

How to Do It for Less

There are millions of people who would benefit from raising their HGH function but who find the cost prohibitive. It would seem, from the junk mail I get, that there are thousands of entrepreneurs out there who have recognized that dilemma and claim to have come up with inexpensive ways to build up your HGH levels without using any HGH at all. This is a worthwhile quest, and one that can be done, but in my opinion not on your own with mail-order products. You can't do this without a doctor's help, preferably one with experience in optimizing hormones. The doctor's role here includes drawing your IGF-1 levels at intervals, writing prescriptions for needed hormones, and evaluating any change in your health status.

Let's look at the most valid and effective treatments that don't require HGH.

DHEA and HGH

The interaction of DHEA and HGH in your body is a good illustration of how intricate your endocrine system is. DHEA is manufactured when your hypothalamus tells your pituitary to tell your adrenal glands to make it—the same as with HGH. And in fact, taking DHEA also makes you produce more IGF-1. It's likely that DHEA makes your body produce more HGH receptor sites on your cells, which would make you more sensitive to the HGH you normally produce. There's no real evidence that DHEA's stimulation of IGF-1 applies to HGH, but there is reason to believe that raising your IGF-1 level gives you many of the same benefits as raising your HGH level.[16]

As you know from the preceding chapter, DHEA has numerous age-defying benefits for your health. In general, it lowers your risk of heart disease, improves your immunity, lifts your mood, and helps prevent cognitive decline. As if those benefits weren't enough, we now know that it helps your body metabolize HGH as well. For all the above reasons, I strongly recommend working with your doctor to optimize your DHEA level before you embark on an HGH or HGH/IGF-1 program.

Stimulating HGH with Amino Acids

Several amino acids stimulate your body to produce HGH; some others may have a similar but less pronounced effect. Let's start by looking at the one we know most about: arginine, an essential amino acid (and one that must come from the diet because your body can't create itself). Arginine has been shown to increase your secretion of growth hormone by blocking the effect of somatostatin.[17]

Studies of the oral dosages needed to have any effect show a wide variation.[18] This may not be a problem, however. Arginine is widely used as a treatment for angina pectoris in dosages of 15 g (about 3 teaspoons). I know from my own experience with angina patients and from the research on the subject that arginine causes virtually no side effects at dosages that high. I have no problem recommending doses of between 5 and 15 g daily and seeing if it causes an improvement in IGF-1 levels.

The nonessential amino acid ornithine is manufactured in

your body from arginine. It is chemically similar to arginine and hence has a very similar effect in the body. The drawback is that while ornithine is roughly twice as effective as arginine, it's also twice as expensive. As with arginine, the best doses are still not really known. For that reason, I prefer to have my patients use arginine and skip the ornithine.

Lysine, another essential amino acid, works synergistically with arginine to boost your HGH output—but only if you're in your twenties. For unknown reasons, the combination doesn't do anything for older adults, even at high doses of 6 g each.[19]

A more promising approach is glutamine, the most abundant amino acid in your body. Glutamine stimulates your body to release growth hormone.[20] Readily available in pills, in capsules, and as a powder, glutamine is inexpensive and very safe. I suggest taking at least 2 g daily at bedtime.

A number of manufacturers now offer arginine and other HGH-stimulating amino acids in combination formulas. Some also offer a sublingual spray that is said to give the same effects with a smaller dose, which is absorbed directly into your bloodstream. Be skeptical about these products—many don't have a large enough dose to be useful. The advertising is sometimes misleading, suggesting that the sprays contain HGH. They do not—HGH is available only with a doctor's prescription.

Hydergine® and HGH

Of all the drugs that raise HGH, the only one I consider prescribing for a patient with a serious HGH deficiency is Hydergine®. Hydergine has been proved to raise HGH levels in elderly patients.[21] It's also often touted as a "smart drug" that can increase your brain power. My European colleagues have long used it with good results for improving cognitive ability in their elderly patients. Studies show Hydergine is quite safe, with a low risk of side effects. There haven't been any long-term studies of its effectiveness for raising HGH levels, but in the short run it definitely helps.

Pumping Up HGH

Exercise stimulates the release of HGH. Any form of exercise is better than none, but weight training seems to give the most dramatic increases in HGH. If you don't think weight training is the right exercise for you, you can get an increase in your HGH levels from taking a brisk walk, riding a bicycle or exercise bike, doing calisthenics, or participating in any other form of exercise that you both enjoy and can do regularly.

Diet and HGH

From reading this book you probably already have a pretty good idea of the easiest way to boost your HGH level while also improving your overall health: lose weight through a low-carbohydrate, high-protein diet. This also just happens to be the diet that is best for enhancing your production of growth hormone.* And speaking of diet, it's time to address the subject of fat.

---

*For more information, please read *Dr. Atkins' New Diet Revolution*.

14

Good Fats and *Really* Bad Fats

I can't go any farther into this book without giving you a clear understanding of the crucial role the right fats play in your age-defying diet. Even more important, I must tell you about the one type of fat you *must* avoid if you are to live to your maximum life span in good health.

Living in our fatphobic society makes many of us dread the mere thought of consuming any sort of dietary fat. In our efforts to avoid these dreaded substances, too many of us then follow the advice of the medical establishment and end up eating far too little of the fats that can help our health and far too high a percentage of the fats that can harm us.

The Good Fats

Despite what the American Heart Association and others would have you believe, you need fat to live and stay healthy. You especially need what are known as essential fatty acids.

Note the use of the word "essential." In scientific as well as common usage, "essential" means just that—something you have to have. Just as vitamins by definition are substances your body can't manufacture and that therefore must be obtained from your food (and supplements, as needed), so too must the essential fatty acids come from your diet. Unfortunately, they often don't. I believe that essential fatty acids are the primary nutrient missing from the American diet.

Essential fatty acids fall into two basic categories: the omega-3 and omega-6 groups. Getting enough of both in the proper balance, as I'll explain a little farther on in this chapter, plays an essential role in maintaining your health.

Let's go a little deeper into the basic concept of essential fatty acids. Your body actually needs to manufacture twenty different fatty acids, all from just two essential fatty acids: omega-3, also known as linolenic acid, and omega-6, also known as linoleic acid.

The omega-3 family of fatty acids can be subdivided into three groups: alpha-linolenic acid (LNA), eicosapentaenoic acid (EPA), and docosahexanoic acid (DHA). In general, omega-3s are found in the leaves and seeds of many plants, in egg yolks, and in cold-water ocean fish such as salmon, herring, tuna, cod, and mackerel. LNA is found in plant foods, especially nuts, soybeans, canola oil, and flaxseed oil. EPA and DHA are found in fish oil.

Similarly, the omega-6 family of fatty acids falls into three groups: gamma-linoleic acid (GLA), arachidonic acid, and dihomo-linoleic acid. Of the three, only GLA and, to a lesser extent, arachidonic acid are really relevant to our discussion here. GLA is found in small amounts in dark-green leafy vegetables, egg yolks, and whole grains and seeds. The only places where it is abundant are in the seeds of plants, especially borage, black currant, and evening primrose, which are not part of the average person's diet.

A third group of fatty acids, the omega-9s, isn't essential, but it is extremely helpful. You've heard of them as the monounsaturated fats, and you probably know that the most widely used source of omega-9 fatty acid is olive oil, also known as oleic acid. It's also found in peanut oil, macadmia nut oil, sesame oil, and other nut oils. Avocados and avocado oil are also excellent dietary sources of monounsaturated fats.

Saturation Point

I'd like to digress a little here to explain a bit more about the structure of fats. I feel it's important to clear up the mystery and misconceptions about fat that many of the American public have.

The biggest confusion relates to the main types of fats: saturated, monounsaturated, and polyunsaturated. Years of agribusiness propaganda have led people to believe that saturated fats must be avoided at all costs and that the more unsaturated a fat is, the better. Let's look more closely at exactly what that means.

Animal fats such as butter and lard are saturated; so are some vegetable oils such as coconut oil and palm oil. Because of their chemical structure, these fats are generally solid at room temperature.

If the chemical structure of the fat is somewhat different, the fat is liquid or very soft at room temperature and is said to be unsaturated. Again, based on chemical structure, unsaturated fats fall into two categories: monounsaturated and polyunsaturated. Olive oil and nut oils are very high in monounsaturated fats; corn oil and safflower oil are very high in polyunsaturated fats.

The prevailing "wisdom" is that eating foods high in saturated fats will lead to increased levels of cholesterol, and that this will inevitably lead to clogged arteries The prevailers go on to say that eating foods high in polyunsaturated fats keeps your arteries clear. It's the simplistic message you hear constantly from every quarter—and it's wrong.

What often gets left out of discussions of fats is that all dietary fats actually contain a mixture of saturated and unsaturated fats. Butter, for instance, is 66 percent saturated fat; the rest is mostly monounsaturated fat. Corn oil is 62 percent polyunsaturated fat, 25 percent monounsaturated fat, and 13 percent saturated fat.

The thing that continually astonishes me about the recommendation to avoid saturated fat is not that I consider that it is based on practically no solid evidence. What really amazes me is how the medical establishment appears to overlook the strong evidence in exactly the opposite direction. The study your doctor is most likely to cite in favor of the saturated fat—heart disease hypothesis is the Framingham Heart Study, which since the 1940s has been following the diets and health of a large group of people living in Framingham, Massachusetts. Here's what Dr. William Castelli, for many years the director of the study, had to say about it in 1992: "In Framingham, Massachusetts, the more saturated fat one ate, the more cholesterol one ate, the more calories one ate, the lower people's serum cholesterol. . . . We found that the people who ate the most cholesterol, ate the most saturated fat, ate the most calories weighed the least and were the most physically active."[1] More recently, in 1997 a major article in the well-regarded *European Heart Journal* was titled "The Low Fat/Low Cholesterol Diet Is Ineffective." The article reviewed all the major studies of diet and heart disease over the last twenty years to prove exactly what the title said it would.[2] That article was followed in 1998 by another meta-analysis of the role of saturated and polyunsaturated fatty acids in cardiovascular disease. The conclusion again was that serious questions have arisen about the role of dietary saturated fats in causing heart disease and the supposed role of polyunsaturated fatty acids in preventing it.[3]

In case all that's not enough to make you start asking your doctor some hard questions, consider a 1999 study that shows how going on a low-fat diet actually increases your chances of heart disease. In this study, 238 healthy men spent several weeks eating a diet that got 40 percent of its calories from fat, then spent an equal amount of time eating a diet that got only 20 to 24 percent of its calories from fat. You might think that while the men were on the low-fat diet, their blood lipid profile would improve. In fact, just the opposite happened. About a third of the men who ate the low-fat diet showed some worrisome lipid changes. They started making more small, dense LDL particles, more triglycerides, and less HDL cholesterol.[4]

Despite all this, your conventional doctor may still be recommending that you eat margarine instead of butter and, more likely, is trying to get you to cut down on red meat and eggs. What he or she could really be doing is assuring that you will be a lifelong patient. Margarine, the fat that agribusiness spends millions a year to advertise, is the worst fat of them all. Why? Because margarine is a trans fat, a fabricated food formed by taking a vegetable oil such as corn, stripping off the essential fatty acids, and processing what's left by forcing additional hydrogen atoms into it. The end product is a fat that's more saturated, which means it is soft or solid at room temperature.

Trans fats, also known as partially hydrogenated vegetable oils, are completely unnatural. Even worse, in the average American diet, trans fats are so widely used that they have largely replaced the essential fatty acids in their natural forms. I'll go into the details of why trans fats are so dangerous toward the end of this chapter. For now, let's get back to why you need essential fatty acids.

What Essential Fatty Acids Do

Your body uses essential fatty acids for a number of important functions. First and foremost, they're used to make eicosanoids and prostaglandins, short-lived, hormonelike substances that regulate many activities in your body. Among other things, eicosanoids and prostaglandins control your blood pressure, control your body temperature, regulate inflammation, swelling, and pain, and are involved in blood clotting, allergic reactions, and making other hormones.

As your body makes the different eicosanoids and prostaglandins, it uses mostly omega-3s for some and mostly omega-6s for others. You can think of the two fatty acids as the brake and accelerator pedals in a car—you need both to drive. If you keep your foot mostly on the accelerator or the brake, however, instead of using both judiciously, you're driving unsafely.

The introduction of vegetable oils made from corn, peanuts, and other sources in the twentieth century has led to a serious imbalance in the amounts of omega-3 and omega-6 fatty acids in the American diet. In general, humans need to take in at least 2 to 3 percent of their fat as omega-6 fatty acids and at least 1 to 1.5 percent as omega-3s. Another way to look at this is that overall you need no more than twice as much omega-6 as omega-3 fatty acids. Unfortunately, the modern American diet has this balance seriously distorted, to the point where we eat many times more omega-6 fatty acids. Historically, in the days before refined vegetable oils, people got their essential fatty acids from whole grains, nuts, vegetables, and egg yolks. Today, the average American consumes large amounts of refined corn, soy, safflower, and canola oils, which are extra-high in omega-6 fatty acids, and relatively little omega-3 fatty acids in the form of fish, egg yolks, nuts and nut oils, unrefined vegetable oils, and whole grains. The resulting imbalance, along with the widespread use of trans fats, is strongly implicated, in my opinion and in the opinion of many others, in today's epidemic levels of heart disease, cancer, inflammatory ailments, autoimmune illnesses, and other chronic, degenerative diseases. Rebalancing your intake of these essential fatty acids is crucial to the age-defying diet.

Omega-3s and Your Heart

Let's take heart disease as one very clear example of the value of omega-3s. As early as 1908, researchers noted that heart disease was unknown among Greenland natives, even though these people subsisted almost entirely on meat. The same lack of heart disease was found when the Greenlanders were studied again in the 1930s. In the 1970s, there was not a single death from heart disease among a group of three thousand natives. To this day, heart disease is very rare among Greenlanders who eat a traditional diet. Why? The native Greenlander diet consists of almost nothing but the meat and blubber from seals and small whales. Because these mammals feed exclusively on cold-water fish, their flesh is very high in omega-3 fatty acids, which in turn confer their protection on the humans who eat them.[5] Native Greenlanders who move to Denmark and begin eating a typical European diet quickly develop levels of heart disease comparable to their Danish neighbors.

The benefits of omega-3 fatty acids to your heart are extremely well documented. They lower triglycerides, lower LDL cholesterol, discourage arterial plaque, act as an anticoagulant to prevent dangerous blood clots, lower high blood pressure, prevent strokes, and perhaps most important of all, prevent sudden death from cardiac arrhythmias.

I could back up all these statements with a discussion of literally hundreds of studies, but let's look just at a couple recent ones. The well-known 1989 Diet and Reinfarction Trial (DART) study of men who had already had a heart attack is a good example. The ones who ate fish at least twice a week had a 29 percent decline in death from any cause compared to the men who didn't change their diets.[6]

A more dramatic study showed that eating fish at least once a week can cut your risk of sudden cardiac death in half. This is borne out by results from the ongoing Physicians' Health Study of more than twenty thousand men. Researchers have been following the diets and health of these male doctors since 1983. Between 1983 and 1994, 133 of the physicians died from sudden cardiac death. The ones who ate fish at least once a week, however, had a 52 percent lower risk of dying that way. Again, the research points to omega-3s as providing protection against fatal heart arrhythmias.[7]

Preventing Cancer with Essential Fatty Acids

Just as eating fish once or twice a week can sharply reduce your chances of dying from heart disease, so too can it reduce your chances of dying from cancer. A major study in Italy that compared ten thousand cancer patients to eight thousand patients with other problems showed that those who ate two or more servings of fish a week had a much lower risk for specific cancers compared to those who ate fish less than once a week. To be precise, the fish eaters had rates of esophageal, stomach, colon, rectum, and pancreatic cancers that were between 30 and 50 percent lower.[8]

Other Benefits of Essential Fatty Acids

The benefits of essential fatty acids go considerably beyond protecting your heart and preventing cancer. Complementary practitioners have long known that fish oil is a valuable treatment for rheumatoid arthritis and other autoimmune diseases such as lupus, multiple sclerosis, and scleroderma. At the Atkins Center we use fish oil as a very effective treatment for Crohn's disease, colitis, and other inflammatory bowel diseases.[9] We also use fish oil to treat skin problems such as atopic eczema and psoriasis. Fish oil has recently been shown to help prevent osteoporosis by inhibiting the production of a prostaglandin that limits bone growth. Adding fish oil to the diet also enhances the activity of insulinlike growth factor 1 (IGF-1), a substance closely related to human growth hormone (HGH)— the miracle age-defyer you read about in Chapter 13. Because IGF stimulates your body to grow and remodel bone, improving your level of it helps prevent osteoporosis.[10]

I've used fish oil as a treatment for mood disorders, particularly depression, with good results for many years. Recently my approach was borne out by a study of thirty patients receiving standard drug therapy for manic depression. Half of the patients took fish oil capsules; the other half took olive oil capsules. Most of the patients on fish oil maintained or improved their mental condition. Most of the patients on olive oil didn't.[11]

The Omega-6s and GLA

I've talked a lot about the omega-3 fatty acids, but let's not forget the omega-6 family. Omega-6 oils, especially arachidonic acid, have been criticized by nutritionists because they are used in the pathways that make prostaglandins that constrict blood vessels, raise blood pressure, and have other undesirable effects. But one omega-6 stands out as nearly essential— gamma-linolenic acid (GLA). Your body needs GLA for making one of its most important natural defenders against degenerative diseases, prostaglandin E_1 (PGE_1). The problem is that the enzyme you use to convert the omega-6s to GLA is often in very short supply in your body. In part, that's because you just naturally make less of it as you get older. A diet high in sugar and partially hydrogenated vegetable oils also tends to suppress your production of the enzyme. The result is a serious shortage of GLA and an increased risk of disease.

At the Atkins Center we use GLA in the form of borage oil or evening primrose oil to help treat a variety of problems. The most common use is for relieving the symptoms of premenstrual tension. The results are generally remarkable—after three months of treatment at 300 mg a day, most women find that the symptoms of PMS, such as irritability, cramps, and breast tenderness, disappear. We also find GLA highly effective for treating arthritis. In fact, this is best documented of all the uses of GLA and has been proved by a number of studies.[12] GLA is very helpful for relieving the joint swelling, morning stiffness, and pain that come with arthritis. It's also useful for some other common problems, such as nerve damage from diabetes and high cholesterol.

Fat, Not Drugs

I hope I have made it clear that altering your balance of omega-3 and omega-6 fatty acids means you can also alter your production of eicosanoids and prostaglandins. Since these chemical messengers control pain and inflammation in your body, by both causing and relieving them, it means that, by altering the balance in the right direction, you can influence your body to produce more of the desirable eicosanoids and prostaglandins and fewer of the undesirable ones. In fact, this is exactly what the two most widely used drugs in medicine, steroids and nonsteroidal anti-inflammatories such as aspirin, do. They inhibit your production of prostaglandins—all prostaglandins, good and bad. How much more sensible it would be to alter only the prostaglandins that are harmful and to do it without powerful drugs and their potentially harmful side effects.

Getting the Benefits of Fatty Acids

By following the age-defying diet I outline in this book, you will remove the two major causes of a deficiency of essential fatty acids. First, you'll be eating far fewer refined carbohydrates and far more eggs, fish, and dark-green leafy vegetables. That means you'll naturally be getting far more omega-3 and omega-6 fatty acids from your diet. Second, you'll be replacing the worthless trans fats in your diet with unrefined natural vegetable oils such as flaxseed oil, olive oil, and the oils of other seeds and nuts. This too will naturally raise your levels of the essential fatty acids and restore them to a more natural balance.

Recent results from the ongoing Nurses' Health Study show how easy it is to add omega-3s to your diet. As part of the study, the diets of more than seventy-six thousand women were tracked for over ten years. During that time, 232 of the women died and 597 developed heart disease. One of the major dietary differences between the women who stayed healthy and those who didn't was how much oil-based salad dressing they ate. Mayonnaise, creamy salad dressing, and oil and vinegar dressings were the most common dietary sources of omega-3 in the study. The women who ate these dressings five or more times a week definitely had healthier hearts than the ones who ate them only rarely.[13]

Here's an excellent example of how fatphobia actually leads inexorably to more heart disease, rather than less. Many people, in their dread of fat of any kind, opt for fat-free salad dressings, even though there's plenty of firm evidence that they should be pouring on dressings rich in these valuable oils instead. You can make your salad dressing even more valuable by adding a tablespoon of flaxseed oil to it. This mild, almost flavorless oil is a very rich source of the essential omega-3, alpha-linolenic acid (LNA).

Another good way to get the age-defying heart protection of omega-3s from your diet is by eating more fish, especially cold-water fish such as salmon, cod, mackerel, sardines, herring, and bluefish. There's no easy way to determine how often you need to eat fish to make a real change in your omega-3 level, although even just twice a week has been shown in various studies to make a measurable difference in successful outcomes. Even if you add fish to your diet, I still recommend taking fish oil supplements just to be sure you're getting enough.

Fish oil is a very effective anticoagulant. Unlike the anticoagulant drug Coumadin, which works by destroying vitamin K and thus keeping your blood from clotting (and also incidentally increasing your risk of osteoporosis because vitamin K plays an important role in bone formation), fish oil keeps the platelets in your blood from clumping together to form a clot. You may be told not to take fish oil or large doses of vitamin E (which works in much the same way) if you are taking Coumadin. The effects are not additive, however, so the warning is overstated.

Just about the only way you can get extra GLA is from capsules of evening primrose oil, borage seed oil, or black currant seed oil. The most inexpensive is borage oil, but the jury is still out on which is the best choice.

To make sure you're getting all the essential fatty acids you need in the right proportions, I recommend that the average person take a mixture of fish oil, flaxseed oil, and borage seed oil, providing 400 mg each of the omega-3 fatty acids LNA, EPA, DHA, and the omega-6 fatty acid GLA—two to four times daily.

Like all oils, essential fatty acids are vulnerable to oxidation, even after you swallow them. You certainly don't want any extra oxidation happening inside your blood vessels. One reason the seal-eating Greenlanders I mentioned above have such low cholesterol levels is that seal oil turns out to be naturally very high in vitamin E and selenium. In fact, Greenlanders who live in the traditional hunting community of Siorapaluk, the northernmost settlement in the world, have selenium levels in their blood that are ten to twenty times higher than those of Europeans or Americans. Free radicals don't have a chance with these people.[14] To get the most benefit from your essential fatty acid supplements, I strongly recommend taking them with a 400-IU capsule of natural vitamin E plus 100 to 200 mcg of selenium.

Adding Essential Fatty Acids to Your Diet

Essential fatty acids are an important component of the age-defying diet. These are easily obtained by substituting unrefined vegetable oils that are mostly monounsaturated or high in omega-3 fatty acids, such as olive oil, nut oils, and flaxseed oil, for the mostly polyunsaturated cooking oils such as corn oil you may now be using. Olive oil is ideal for high-temperature cooking such as sautéing. It is also excellent for salad dressings and homemade mayonnaise. Flaxseed oil is a mild, almost flavorless oil that is extremely high in alpha-linolenic acid. Add a spoonful to salad dressings and the like, but don't heat it—you'll oxidize the oil. Nut oils, such as walnut oil, add a rich flavor to salad dressings.

Commercial cooking oils are heavily processed at high temperatures in harsh chemicals so a lot of their nutritional value is destroyed long before they end up in your shopping cart. I strongly urge you to purchase cold-pressed, unrefined cooking oils at your health food store. To prevent oxidation, the oils should be stored in the refrigerator in opaque bottles.

Another good way to get extra omega-3s in your diet is to go a little nuts! Eat a handful of walnuts, macadamias, almonds, pecans, hazelnuts, or even peanuts (which technically are legumes, not nuts) every day. Going back to the Nurses' Health Study, researchers recently found that the women who ate nuts regularly had a 32 percent lower risk of having a nonfatal heart attack and were 39 percent less likely to die of a heart attack than those who never or rarely consumed nuts.[15] The amount of nuts needed to provide the protection was low—only five ounces a week. Similar results from the Physicians' Health Study suggest that frequent nut consumption has the same benefits for men. The fatty acids in the nuts help to lower LDL cholesterol and triglycerides while leaving HDL cholesterol at the same level or even raising it. I especially recommend nuts high in monounsaturated fat such as macadamias, hazelnuts, and pecans. Peanuts are good too, but avoid most commercial peanut butters, which can be loaded with trans fats and extra sugar.

The Mediterranean Diet

All this discussion of the different types of fats brings us directly to the benefits—alleged and real—of the Mediterranean diet. As you probably know, the heart-protective Mediterranean diet is what the natives of Greece and Italy eat—a diet high in fresh fruits and vegetables, whole grains, fish, olive oil, and red wine. The nutritional establishment has seized on what's relatively missing from the Mediterranean diet—red meat, butter, and dairy products—and proclaimed this as proof that a high-carbohydrate, low-fat diet is indeed the most healthful way to eat. What they don't quite see is that the two things that make the Mediterranean diet healthful are the dearth of refined carbohydrates and the high amount of essential fatty acids in it from fish fat, olive oil, and nut oils. In fact, a recent study has shown that the monounsaturated fats in the Mediterranean diet help protect you against age-related memory loss. The higher your consumption of olive oil, which is a very rich source of monounsaturated oleic acid (omega-9 fatty acid), the better protected you are.[16]

Trans Fats: The Worst

To avoid the dangerous effects of trans fats, you need to understand what they are. As I discussed near the start of this chapter, trans fats are polyunsaturated vegetable oils that have been processed to make them solid at room temperature—these fats are known as partially hydrogenated oils. Heating polyunsaturated vegetable oils, as you do when you deep-fry foods in corn, safflower, peanut, and other common oils, is another way to produce trans fats.

Partially hydrogenated oils are used extensively in processed foods, especially baked goods. To see what I mean, go to the cookie aisle of your supermarket and read the ingredients on just about any package, even the so-called whole-grain breads and the super-premium cookies. Partially hydrogenated vegetable oil is sure to be one of the top three or four ingredients, right after the enriched white flour. You'll also find this stuff in all sorts of other prepared foods, including prepared entrees, mayo, salad dressings, candy bars, potato chips, and lots more. And of course, margarine, even the low-fat kind, is by definition nothing but a stick or tub of trans fats.

Any food fried in polyunsaturated oil—the french fries at your favorite fast-food restaurant, for example—is basically being fried in trans fats, probably made from soybean oil. Instead of being better for you than food fried in saturated fats such as lard, tallow, or palm oil, these foods are actually worse. In fact, if you need a second reason, beyond sugar and flour, for why Americans today are fatter than ever, trans fats are it.

What makes these molecular misfits so dangerous is the way they raise your LDL cholesterol, triglycerides, and lipoprotein(a) levels and lower your HDL cholesterol—the worst possible combination of lipid changes and the surest markers we have of almost certain cardiovascular disease sooner rather than later in life.[17] Instead of wrongly blaming saturated fat from animal foods for atherosclerosis, the finger should be pointed straight at trans fats.*

---

*In fact, it was all the way back in 1956 when a researcher named Dr. Ancel Keys claimed that the trans fats in partially hydrogenated vegetable oils were the culprits. Dr Keys went on to be the author of the 1966 Seven Countries study that provided the "proof" that high saturated-fat consumption in a population correlates directly to high rates of heart disease. This study, felt to be deeply flawed by the selection of seven nations chosen to prove a point from the contradictory data of twenty nations, has since become the touchstone of the fatphobic public policy now being foisted on the American populace.

Trans fats not only displace the natural fats and oils in the diet that provide essential fatty acids, they also block your uptake and use of the essential fatty acids you do manage to take in. What happens then? The trans fats are deposited in parts of your cell membranes that should really be filled by essential fatty acids. This quite literally gums up the works. Aside from weakening the integrity of the cell membranes, you also have trouble making the enzyme that converts essential fatty acids into the other fatty acids you need.[18]

Also, trans fats aggravate the problem I consider the major life shortener—they make you put out more insulin than normal in response to blood glucose, while making your red blood cells less responsive to insulin.[19]

The medical establishment, backed up by the massive American food-processing industry, has in my view, not recognised the glaring dangers of trans fats ever since the first evidence was published in the 1950s. Numerous other studies have been published since then, particularly by the distinguished fat researcher Mary G. Enig, Ph.D. Recently even the establishment's medical press has published major studies pointing out the dangers of trans fats and even admitting that earlier recommendations to eat margarine instead of butter were incorrect.[20] The word still hasn't seeped out to conventional doctors—or if it has, they've decided to ignore it. Most still parrot the party line that saturated fats are the culprit. Don't believe it for a minute. The lack of trans fats in the American diet is a major reason why heart disease was practically nonexistent before 1910, when margarine was introduced as a cheap and "healthy" substitute for butter. Crisco, a partially hydrogenated vegetable shortening, was introduced in 1911. By 1950, annual butter consumption dropped from eighteen pounds per person to just ten, but margarine consumption went up from two pounds per person to eight. In 1909, the average American ate less than two grams a day of liquid vegetable oils. In 1993, that number had jumped to more than thirty grams. Combine the switch from animal fats to liquid vegetable oils with the fact that refined carbohydrate intake escalated at the same time and you have a convincing explanation for the increase in heart attack deaths from three thousand in 1930 to half a million just thirty years later.

Today, based on results from the Nurses' Health Study, your risk of a heart attack is nearly double the average if you get just 2 percent of your calories from the trans fats in doughnuts, french fries, margarine, and similar foods. Unfortunately, 2 percent of your calories from trans fats is almost certainly on the low side for a typical American today. Fat expert Mary Enig thinks that the typical intake of trans fats is much higher. On the basis of solid evidence, she believes that of the total fat in the diet of the average American today, about 11 percent is trans fats. That works out to be closer to 4 percent of the average American's total daily calories.[21]

Trans fats are ubiquitous and insidious, yet the amounts in prepared foods aren't required to be listed on the labels. Many fast foods are practically nothing but trans fats. A large order of fries at a fast-food restaurant, for instance, could easily contain nearly seven grams of trans fats—but the restaurant proudly proclaims that the fries are cholesterol free! Fortunately, there is a strong movement afoot at the FDA to force manufacturers to list the amount of trans fats on their labels separately from the amount of saturated fat. I hope that the adoption of this regulation will soon take place reflecting a welcome common sense decision by the FDA.

I've learned over the years that most of my patients and readers have plenty of common sense—that's why they're interested in their health. Well, it's just common sense to do everything you can to avoid getting sick. In the next chapter, I'll tell you about lifelong ways to boost your immunity.

15

Build Your Immunity

It is just possible that the upbeat major message of this book—"It's your diet"—may not be enough. Your diet is central to defying age and preventing many chronic illnesses, but it's becoming increasingly clear that to truly defy age, we must consider factors beyond the diet, the most important of which is stress. There can be no question that a major key to a successful age-defying program is to develop the most powerful immune defenses we can. Diet, of course, plays a central role in boosting your immunity, but we must also pay careful attention to vitanutrients and even lifestyle to achieve the most resilient immune system possible.

Eating for Immunity

Whenever I put a patient onto a low-carbohydrate, high-protein diet, I schedule a follow-up visit for a few months later. At that visit, my patients almost always say things like, "Doctor, I haven't been sick once since I went on your diet" or "Doctor, that nagging infection I had cleared up just a few days after I started the diet." I'm never surprised to hear this—indeed, the only surprise would be if someone told me the opposite, that he or she had gotten sick.

There's no question that the age-defying diet improves your immunity, but how? Your immune system is a very complex and interconnected arrangement of many different kinds of immune cells and chemical messengers, including hormones, eicosanoids, and enzymes. To function efficiently and produce all its component parts, your immune system needs a good supply of high-quality protein and crucial vitanutrients.

If you take in all the protein and nutrients your immune system needs, however, and still also take in high levels of carbohydrates, you won't get the full benefit of increased immunity. The high level of carbohydrates in your diet is almost certain to lead to high levels of glucose in your blood, which in turn will cause you to release large amounts of insulin—and high levels of insulin can severely depress your immune system. By keeping your blood sugar and insulin levels as low as possible, you keep your immune system at a high level of readiness.

Sugar in itself also has a severely depressing effect on your immune system. Eating sweet foods of any sort interferes with the ability of your white blood cells to attack and destroy invading pathogens. The negative effect of just one glass of soda pop or even orange juice can linger for more than twelve hours. In addition, sugar lowers your body's ability to produce antibodies, the chemical messengers that recognize invaders and sound the alert that mobilizes your white blood cells to attack them.[1]

Another crucial element of your diet as it relates to immunity is your intake of essential fatty acids. I've discussed the importance of EFAs at length in the previous chapter, so here

I'll just remind you that the balance of omega-3 and omega-6 fatty acids is very important for your production of the chemical messengers—hormones and eicosanoids—that tell your immune system what to do. If the balance is tipped too far in favor of the omega-6 EFAs, as it often is among people who eat a typical American diet, the pathways that create the chemical messengers won't function properly. The messages will be garbled or may not get through at all, with the result that your immune system falters and functions far below peak efficiency.

Your body also needs some support against your immune system. Let me explain that apparent contradiction. When your white blood cells (lymphocytes) fend off an invading pathogen, as they do quite literally millions of times a day in a healthy person, they generate large quantities of free radicals in the process. If you're sick, your immune system will be generating free radicals at a rate that is orders of magnitude higher. To protect yourself against the damage from the excess free radicals, you need a diet high in natural antioxidants, as well as supplementary antioxidant vitanutrients.

There's one final factor to consider for strengthening your immunity. You've probably noticed that you're more likely to get sick when you're under stress. That's explainable. Stress produces the hormone cortisol, and cortisol can slow your immune system or shut it down altogether by blocking your production of chemical messengers. In earlier times when life was simpler (say, a hundred thousand years ago), shutting down your immune system occasionally while your body's energies were diverted to fighting off a cave bear did no lasting harm.

Cortisol levels rise naturally as we get older. Combine that with the constant high stress of life at the start of the twenty-first century, and it's quite likely that your cortisol level is continuously high, with a correspondingly depressing effect on your immunity. As I discussed in Chapter 12, lowering your overall cortisol level also plays an important role.

Immunity and Cancer

So far I've been discussing your immune system as if the only thing it does is protect you against illness caused by infectious agents. Your immune system, however, has an even more important function: It protects you against cancer. Your immune cells, especially the ones known as NK (natural killer) cells and T lymphocytes, and the antitumor chemicals (cytokines) such as interferon that the lymphocytes manufacture, constantly patrol your body on the lookout for your own defective cells. These are cells whose genetic material has been damaged, making them potentially or actually cancerous. Cell damage of this sort is far from unusual in your body—it happens all the time, generally as a result of free radical damage. Your body's natural antioxidant defenses keep the damage down, but you must rely on continuous surveillance from a strong, efficient immune system to detect and destroy those cells that do get damaged before they begin to multiply uncontrollably.

Vitanutrients for Immunity

Your body's primary defense against invading pathogens is your skin and your epithelial cells—the linings of your organs, including your respiratory and intestinal tracts. If these are weak, harmful infectious agents can enter more easily. If an infectious agent does make it past your epithelial defenses, your internal defense systems—the various kinds of white blood cells, antibodies, and chemical messengers—take over. All aspects of your immune system are on constant patrol to detect not just invading pathogens but also defective and cancerous cells within your body.

To maintain a strong defense, you need to make sure not

only that you get adequate levels of protein from your diet but also that your intake of supporting vitanutrients is high. Let's look at the vitanutrients that are most important to building and maintaining your immune system. I'll discuss each one separately.*

Vitamin A: Infection Fighter

One of the most important immune-supportive vitanutrients is vitamin A. When vitamin A was discovered early in the twentieth century, it was called the anti-infective agent, because it's so important for keeping your epithelial cells moist and flexible. In general, vitamin A reinforces your immune system's ability to resist infections. It's particularly helpful for protecting you against "stomach bugs" by keeping the mucous membranes that line your intestinal tract strong and impermeable to germs.

If you do get sick or get an infection, large doses of vitamin A can do a lot to clear it up quickly. Taking 50,000 IU the moment you feel a cold coming, along with some extra vitamin C and zinc, can help keep the illness mild and short; it may even stop it in its tracks. It's also very effective for treating sinus infections. And don't worry about the high dose when it's given as a one-shot deal. You'd have to take a dose that high for a week or more to have a harmful effect.

Vitamin A is useful for treating a current illness or infection, but for overall immune enhancement I prefer to see my patients take vitamin A builders in the form of mixed carotenoid supplements. Research has shown that taking 50,000 IU of beta-carotene daily can cause a significant improvement in

*For detailed information, please see *Dr. Atkins' Vita-Nutrient Solution.*

immune function.[2] In particular, beta-carotene supplements improve the activity of your natural killer cells, which attack viruses and tumor cells and play an important role in preventing cancer.[3] Supplements containing mixed carotenoids, which contain mostly beta-carotene but also other carotenes, give your immune system a boost and also give you all the other benefits of carotenoids (see Chapter 10 for more on the value of carotenoids).

The B Complex Vitamins

The complete B complex vitamins are essential for creating white blood cells. You need all of them in the proper balance to do this efficiently. The absence of one or the overabundance of another throws off the whole delicate balance, with a corresponding reduction in your body's ability to fight off illness. It's hard to say, then, that any one B vitamin is more important than the others, but even so, I must make a special case for vitamin B_6, also known as pyridoxine. This vitanutrient is crucial for making adequate numbers of infection-fighting T cells.[4] I strongly recommend that you get between 100 and 250 mg a day to keep your immunity high.

Vitamin C and the Common Cold

Because you're reading this book, you may already have an interest in complementary medicine. In that case, you've probably experienced for yourself the way large doses of vitamin C can shorten the duration of a cold or flu. For those of you who need some convincing that this simple, inexpensive, safe vitanutrient really helps, let's look at how it works. More than twenty different studies tell us that the primary reason vitamin C fights colds so well is that it boosts the overall function of your immune system, especially the various types of white blood cells. These cells work best when they're saturated with as much vitamin C as they can hold. Illness depletes their vitamin C levels; supplements build it back up again.[5]

Cutting off respiratory illnesses such as colds and flus quickly becomes even more important as you age, because these illnesses are more likely to turn into bronchitis or even pneumonia in older adults. Taking just 1,000 mg a day of extra vitamin C could cut the duration of your cold by about 20 percent—in practice, you'll get better a day or so sooner.[6]

Space does not permit me to go into the many dozens of studies that show how vitamin C protects you against cancer. The overall idea, however, is that vitamin C works against cancer chiefly for two reasons. First, it is a very powerful antioxidant, which means it neutralizes free radicals before they have the chance to do the sort of damage that initiates cancer. Second, your T lymphocytes, which are one of your body's main defenses against cancer, need plenty of vitamin C to function at peak levels. In short, vitamin C is widely regarded as the most powerful anticarcinogenic nutrient known.[7] It's borne out by epidemiological studies of eighty-eight different populations worldwide.[8] Need I say more?

Vitamin E for Excellent

One of the more interesting recent pieces of vitanutrient research is the "discovery" that vitamin E enhances immunity. This has been a well-known fact among complementary practitioners for years, but perhaps now the information will trickle down to mainstream medicine, where this sort of knowledge is badly needed. The most recent study looked at the effect of vitamin E on the immune systems of eighty-eight healthy older adults. Half took supplemental vitamin E; half took a placebo. After three months, the people taking vitamin E had measurably higher levels of T cells; after six months, their ability to produce infection-fighting antibodies was markedly higher. The best results came from the group that took a mere 200 IU daily.[9]

If vitamin C and vitamin E are both good for immunity, what happens when you combine them? You get even better immunity. A recent study showed that combined supplementation with 1,000 mg of vitamin C and 800 IU of vitamin E for just thirty days increased several parameters of immune function in all older adults, but it was especially effective for inactive older men.[10]

Let me just remind you that the results of the Third National Health and Nutrition Examination Survey (NHANES III) showed that almost 30 percent of American adults have low blood levels of vitamin E.[11] These people are setting themselves up not just for avoidable infectious disease but also avoidable heart disease and cancer. Doses of vitamin E of up to 3,200 IU daily are very safe, but you don't need to take that much. I generally recommend 400 to 800 IU of natural (not synthetic) vitamin E a day.

Zinc for Immune System Zing

Your body needs zinc to manufacture more than two hundred different enzymes. No zinc, no enzymes—including enzymes that are crucial to proper immune system function. Specifically, you need zinc to manufacture white blood cells and support the activity of your neutrophils, T cells, and natural killer

(NK) cells. These are the lymphocytes that kill cancer cells and fight off infections. Much of the zinc in your body, in fact, is tied up in these cells. Enzymes and other proteins made with zinc play a central role in cell growth and differentiation in your body. They're also important for regulating normal cell death—a sort of cellular suicide, where your immune system orders defective cells to self-destruct. If the orders don't get through, the defective cells may divide uncontrollably instead—in other words, they become cancerous.

The most popular use of zinc today is in lozenges as a way to fend off colds and flu. If you start using the lozenges as soon as you feel the first symptoms, you could cut down cold symptoms from an average of about a week to just four days.[12] For fighting colds, I generally recommend sugarless lozenges made with zinc gluconate with glycine. Let the lozenge dissolve slowly in your mouth; don't chew it. Adults can use a lozenge once every few hours for up to two days—don't take more than twelve lozenges in a day. Make sure each lozenge contains at least 22 mg of zinc. Anything less won't do you much good.

Zinc helps wounds heal, including surgical ones. If you must have an operation, taking zinc supplements for several weeks both before and after the surgery will help you heal faster with less chance of infection. And if you have a wound that's not healing well, it could be that you're low on zinc.

Zinc also acts to improve the action of your thymus gland. This is a small organ in your neck just above your breastbone. The thymus is crucial to your health, because it makes some of the hormones that tell your immune system what to do. Your thymus gland is quite large when you're an infant, but by the time you reach your teens, it has naturally shrunk quite a bit. By the time you're forty, your thymus may have shrunk so much that it can't really be found anymore. And by the time you're in your fifties, your thymus is practically nonexistent.

Although a certain amount of thymus shrinking is considered normal, you certainly don't want it disappearing on you. One way to keep your thymus gland going is to make sure you get plenty of zinc. It's also possible that taking zinc supplements can revitalize your thymus and get it working again. (I'll expand on other ways to improve thymus function below.)

Even though the basic daily zinc requirement is only about 15 mg for men and 12 mg for women, a distressingly large number of adults, especially older adults, are deficient.[13] A recent study of older adults in Italy found that taking 25 mg of zinc sulfate daily for three months led to an improvement in the overall status of their immune systems, based on their T cell count. To avoid a deficiency and get the benefit of extra zinc, I suggest taking 25 mg a day.[14]

Ironclad Protection

Iron gets a good press, but it poses problems for your immune defenses. True, iron deficiency is one of the most common nutritional deficiencies in America. It's fairly widespread among older adults, especially those who live on a high-carbohydrate, high-fiber, low- or no-meat diet. These people don't get much iron from their food, and the iron they do get is bound up in the fiber and often passes through their body without being absorbed. That means you should have your doctor test your blood for iron deficiency, and, if you find it, to treat the problem by adding red meat to your diet.

But it is iron's flip side that can be dangerous. Here's how. Excess iron in your system can lead to increased oxidation—you quite literally rust from it. Iron can damage your antioxidant protection system. Iron can also feed the growth of tumor cells and harmful bacteria. If you're suffering from an illness or infection, especially if it's affecting your gastrointestinal tract, stay away from inorganic iron supplements. You can best correct any anemia tendency with the natural iron that comes from red meat, chicken, and fish. This form, called heme iron, can't build up in your body and isn't vulnerable to oxidation.

Nonetheless, too little iron, it turns out, is much riskier than too much. According to a study of all-cause death rates of older adults, men and women with the highest blood levels of iron had 38 percent and 28 percent lower death rates, respectively.[15]

Supplementing Your Immunity with DHEA

In Chapter 12 I talked extensively about the many virtues of DHEA. Here let me briefly review how important DHEA is to your immune health. The mother hormone DHEA improves your production of antibodies. It also boosts the action of the various types of white blood cells that attack and kill viruses and cancer cells, including monocytes, natural killer cells, and T lymphocytes. In short, taking DHEA can restore your immune system function to the level you enjoyed in your twenties and thirties, when most people are at their healthiest.

Herbal Immune Boosters

At the Atkins Center we are very much opposed to the sort of indiscriminate antibiotic use that is widely practiced by conventional physicians. This dangerous practice is the primary cause of the new epidemic of antibiotic-resistant pathogens. On the level of the individual patient, we find that antibiotics often cause as many problems as they solve. Rather than use antibiotics, whenever possible and prudent I prefer to help the patient's own immune system overcome the infectious organisms. To help the immune system work its hardest, I prescribe the vitanutrients discussed above, along with a number of valuable herbal supplements that are proven immune enhancers.

First and foremost among the immune-enhancing herbs is garlic. Rich in selenium and germanium, two trace minerals that are important for manufacturing immune cells, garlic is a broad-spectrum antimicrobial that is quite effective for destroying bacteria, including some that have become antibiotic resistant. Garlic is also an effective antioxidant, so taking it is almost certain to prove helpful in managing any infectious disease. Overall, garlic stimulates your immune system, with a particularly beneficial effect on your production of natural killer cells.

To get the immune-enhancing benefits of garlic, it's preferable to take 2,400 to 3,200 mg daily. Eating that amount of the herb might upset your digestion, to say nothing of the powerful garlic breath you'd develop. I personally prefer to eat the garlic in food, but taking odorless, tasteless extract of dried garlic, in capsule or liquid form, is an acceptable option.

After garlic, my next favorite herb for immunity is ginseng. Overall, ginseng is valuable as an adaptogen, an herb that helps the body adjust to stress. Ginseng is generally used to improve mental and physical stamina, to the point that its value as an immune enhancer is sometimes overlooked. In fact, however, placebo-controlled studies tell us that taking ginseng can shorten the duration of colds and flu, and may even help protect you against getting them.[16] The German Commission E, which evaluates herbs for the German government, considers ginseng a nonspecific immunostimulant, but there's some good evidence that ginseng works to stimulate your production of natural killer cells.[17] Animal studies on a pneumonia-causing organism confirm ginseng's ability to fight bacteria.[18] Of course, ginseng is also a powerful antioxidant that has been shown to prevent lipid peroxidation. It also quenches hydroxyl, the most dangerous of the free radicals.[19]

I often suggest daily ginseng supplements to patients who are under a lot of stress or whose immunity is low. Look for a standardized supplement that contains 5 to 10 percent ginsenoides. I generally recommend 100 to 200 mg one to three times daily. The effects could take a couple of weeks or even longer to be felt. If you think ginseng is making you feel irritable or anxious or is disturbing your sleep, try cutting back on the dosage.

My final favorite herb for enhancing immunity is echinacea. This herb, made from the roots of the purple coneflower, was well known to the Plains Indians, who introduced it to Europeans hundreds of years ago. Echinacea reinforces your natural immune defenses. It's very useful not just for preventing illness, especially colds and upper respiratory infections, but also for speeding your recovery time.

During cold and flu season, I recommend taking two to three capsules a day of freeze-dried echinacea powder as a preventive. If you do get sick, taking six to eight capsules a day will help you feel better sooner.

Glutamine: Fueling Your Immune System

The most abundant amino acid in your body is glutamine. It's also perhaps the most valuable for helping you recover from illness and injury and for keeping your immune system working at peak efficiency.

Glutamine is the primary source of energy for your immune system. You always need lots of it, but when you're sick or have an infection, your immune system goes into overdrive and needs extra fuel. If it doesn't get enough glutamine, the system will sputter along and won't be able to knock out the infectious agents very well. You'll end up being sicker for longer. The same is true for recovering from an injury, such as a bad cut or burn, and from surgery. You need plenty of glutamine to heal the wound and nourish your immune system.[20]

For immune support, I recommend anywhere from 5 to 20 g of glutamine a day. If you're fighting an infectious illness or healing from an injury or surgery, you can increase to as much as 40 g a day.

Thymus Support

As I mentioned earlier, your thymus gland is the organ of immunity, yet it shrinks as you get older. Thymus extracts can be given to compensate. I am quite happy using an over-the-counter product derived from a culture of thymus cells called thymus protein A. I prescribe it for cancer patients and those with debilitating chronic infections.

It also makes sense to stimulate the thymus into greater output of the hormones that the gland is responsible for making.

One possible way to stimulate your thymus is with melatonin, a hormone secreted by your pineal gland. (I discussed melatonin at length in Chapter 13.) Some recent research indicates that melatonin may help reinvigorate your thymus gland—and also your spleen and bone marrow, both of which are crucial for the production of lymphocytes. Your thymus, spleen, and bone marrow cells all appear to have receptor sites for melatonin on them. We also know that melatonin may help reverse age-related declines in your production of antibodies. So far, some encouraging studies on why you have melatonin receptors on your thymus, and what they do, have been done largely on lab rodents. The animals given melatonin made more antibodies and other immune system chemicals.[21] Does this mean melatonin can improve human immunity? The evidence isn't in yet, but I believe it can. Because melatonin also has other benefits as a potent antioxidant, I recommend taking it for that purpose—there may well be immune benefits as well.

If you've been doing the things I recommend in this chapter and yet you still have frequent minor illnesses, there's a good chance that your body is overloaded with toxins that are weakening your immune defenses. In the next chapter, let's look at techniques that can remove the toxins and restore your health.

16

Detoxify Your Body

A legacy of the twentieth century we are very unlikely to shake off in the twenty-first is our massive, continuous exposure to toxins from our environment. There's no way to avoid them. Every day, the typical American is exposed to a huge number of potentially toxic substances: automobile exhaust fumes, smog, household cleaning products, tobacco smoke, paint fumes, chlorinated water, lead, cadmium, mercury, and other heavy metals, pesticides, food additives, prescription and nonprescription drugs, and much more.

Your body's waste-removal systems were never designed for the sort of toxic onslaught that most of us now experience every day. For example, take the chemical element cadmium. Used in many industrial processes and also found in cigarette smoke, cadmium is something humans were never exposed to until the past couple of centuries. You have no natural detoxification pathway in your body for removing cadmium. Once it enters your body, it stays there, possibly triggering lung cancer and other diseases.

Toxins and Aging

Exposure to toxins, whether naturally from the ultraviolet radiation of the sun, or unnaturally from smog and other industrial pollutants, is a major factor in aging. Why? Because toxins create free radicals—and as you certainly know by now, damage from free radicals is the underlying cause of most of the diseases of aging, and of aging itself.

Are You Poisoning Yourself?

Another source of toxins in your body could very well be your own digestive system. If you can't eliminate toxins well, your overall health will suffer, and any health problems you do have will be accentuated if the intestinal tract accumulates toxic waste products. Of even more concern are toxins created in your intestinal tract by the presence of a yeast overgrowth, also known as candidiasis. This problem has achieved such epidemic proportions that I must devote the next few pages to discussing its causes and treatments.

Ordinarily, your intestines contain trillions of bacteria that are essential to your digestion. They are a vital part of the process that breaks down your food into nutrients you can absorb. Often, however, those beneficial bacteria get crowded out by an overgrowth of the yeastlike organism called *Candida albicans*, which is a normal resident of the large intestine. What causes this to happen? A host of medical and dietary abuses. The major cause is the use of antibiotics, which kill off the beneficial bacteria that otherwise hold the growth of the yeast in check. Yeast also overgrows from the use of hormones such as prednisone, body-building steroids, and birth-control pills.

Poor diet plays a major role by itself. The chief culprit by far is too much sugar in the diet, followed closely by foods that are high in natural sugar, such as fruit, honey, fruit juice, and milk. Alcohol, food additives, food intolerances (especially lactose or gluten intolerance), insufficient stomach acid, and emotional stress all can trigger yeast overgrowth. An often overlooked factor in yeast overgrowth is the role of untreated bacterial infections and parasites.

There can be no question that the most likely cause of yeast overgrowth is either antibiotic abuse or overconsumption of sugar—and as often as not, the two in combination. In fact, yeast overgrowth is often a key ingredient in the larger disease picture of conditions such as chronic fatigue syndrome, frequently recurring infections, Crohn's disease, colitis, and irritable bowel syndrome. It's also a major contributor to food intolerances.

Approximately one in three patients at the Atkins Center is found to have a yeast overgrowth. The diagnosis is most reliably made by a blood test that measures for elevated IgA or IgM antibodies to candida. The diagnosis can also be inferred by a variety of symptoms, especially lower intestinal gas and bloating, frequent bouts of diarrhea and constipation, decreased resistance to infection, chronic fatigue syndrome, "brain fog," recurrent bladder infections, and thrush, a whitish plaque in the mouth and throat. Joint pain, fatigue, and depression are also common symptoms. Yeast overgrowth is also strongly associated with arthritis.[1]

When you have a yeast overgrowth, the yeast organisms produce some seventy-nine different toxins, including formaldehyde and acetaldehyde, which is exactly the same toxin you get from drinking alcohol. Acetaldehyde is responsible for the "brain fog" that is often associated with candidiasis. And from the age-defying standpoint, bear in mind that yeast overgrowth in the large intestine produces massive amounts of cell-damaging free radicals. The toxins from harmful bacteria in the gut are also a possible cause of Alzheimer's disease and Parkinson's disease.[2] By maintaining a good balance of beneficial bacteria in your intestines, you prevent the buildup of metabolic poisons that may be behind these and other diseases associated with aging.

Yeast in your intestines lives on sugar, so the first step in curing an overgrowth is simply to deprive yeast of its favorite food. At the Atkins Center, we start by putting candidiasis patients on a low-carbohydrate, sugar-free diet that eliminates all simple sugars as well as all cured, salted, fermented, or yeast-containing foods such as cheese, vinegar, alcohol, and bread. Of course, patients also avoid any foods to which they have a known intolerance.

We use food-derived therapies such as grapefruit seed extract, oil of oregano, caprylic acid, undecenylic acid, or olive leaf extract to kill off the yeast and any parasites. This is a very effective approach that I believe is more appropriate than Diflucan®, the usual drug prescribed for candidiasis. Here I must mention one side effect of the treatment. For the first few days, patients may sometimes feel worse instead of better. That's because the yeast are dying off in large numbers, which makes your intestines temporarily more toxic. If you feel a lot worse or if the symptoms persist, call your doctor. The symptoms of die-off can be controlled by using these effective natural agents in smaller doses, but in a way, they're worth experiencing for the improvement that follows soon after. The results are little short of miraculous for some patients—their health and energy are restored after years of chronic tiredness, digestive upsets, frequent illness, and poor mental function.

The most important therapy while you are on the antiyeast diet is to restore a healthy balance of beneficial bacteria (called probiotics) in your intestines. Three friendly bacteria strains are used to reinoculate your digestive tract: acidophilus (lactobacillus), bifidus, and bulgaricus. Many patients take capsules containing five hundred thousand spores of each; others take each probiotic by the tablespoon (they're tasteless). The doses may seem huge, but remember that the healthy gut contains around nine times more probiotic organisms than there are cells in your body—in other words, a normal, healthy person has trillions of bacteria in the small and large intestine.

Treating a yeast overgrowth is a long-term project. It could easily take two to four months to evict the yeast and restore a healthy balance.

Once that balance is restored, Atkins Center patients switch over to the intestinal repair part of the program. We use a variety of vitanutrients to restore the integrity of your intestinal walls and build up your ability to resist unfriendly bacteria, including pantethine, glutamine, N-acetyl-cysteine, essential fatty acids, and gamma oryzanol (rice bran oil). We also add fiber in the form of psyllium husks, which helps food move through your system quickly and regularly. This keeps the yeast from gaining a foothold again. The repair process can take another two to four months.

Probiotics and fiber are so valuable for reducing your body's toxic load that I recommend them for everyone, not just as a treatment for candidiasis. By maintaining a healthy bacterial balance in the intestines, you significantly reduce your liver's workload and let it concentrate on removing the unavoidable toxins.

As a part of my age-defying program, I suggest taking weekly or twice-weekly probiotic supplements of acidophilus, bifidus, and bulgaricus. One 500-mg capsule of each on an empty stomach may be enough—as long as you get a high-quality probiotic that truly contains what the label states. In addition, be sure that you get at least 7 to 10 g of fiber in your diet daily. Use psyllium husks as a way to get the extra fiber if you can't get enough from the vegetables in your diet—a daily dose of one tablespoon stirred into at least eight ounces of pure water should do the trick.

Reducing Your Exposure

In today's society we must simply accept that we are inevitably exposed to numerous toxins all the time. The most we can hope to do, short of moving to Alaska and living in a log cabin far from civilization, is to minimize our exposure and maximize our defenses.

To minimize your exposure, start by considering the water you drink. Your household water is probably chlorinated and fluoridated by your municipality and may also be picking up copper and lead as it passes through metal pipes on its way to you. (I'll talk about just how dangerous lead is to you a little later in this chapter.) The chlorine and fluoride are added to kill bacteria—which means they kill *all* bacteria, including the beneficial bacteria in your intestines. Even worse, tap water may have been contaminated along the way with dangerous pathogens, such as *E. coli* or cryptosporidium, that chlorine doesn't kill. These pathogens can cause severe stomach upsets. Indeed, children, the elderly, and anyone with a compromised immune system can die from them. I strongly recommend that you install household water filters on all the taps in your home. I recommend using the ceramic filter type, which is reasonably priced, easy to install, and lasts a long time. When pure filtered water isn't available, stick to bottled water whenever possible. (Although, I must say, bottling does not always provide assurance that the water is not contaminated.)

The very air you breathe can be a major source of toxins. You might think that the problem of air pollution isn't so bad if you don't live in a city that regularly has smog alerts, but that's not necessarily the case. At the Atkins Center we frequently see patients who complain that they often get headaches, dizziness, anxiety, and "brain fog" at the office. They put it down to the stress of their jobs. My first question is, "Do you work in a sealed office building, the kind where you can't open the windows?" If the answer is yes, as it often is, we've often found the root of the problem. It isn't stress—these people are perfectly capable of doing their jobs well. It's their environment. The sealed building typical of a suburban office park is a sinkhole for all the chemicals that are found in today's offices. Toxic fumes from carpeting, paint, plastic furniture, copying machines, solvents, cleaning fluids, and many more substances are trapped inside the building, especially if the ventilation system is poor, as it often is. You end up breathing them in, along with all the germs exhaled by your fellow workers. It's not surprising that "sick building syndrome" sometimes leads to epidemics of chronic fatigue, headaches, dizziness, rashes, and other symptoms among the workers in an office.

You can reduce the toxic level of the air around you by insisting that your work environment be properly ventilated, as federal law requires. At home, and if possible at the office, use HEPA air filters, which are very good for removing toxins, particulates, and allergens such as mold spores from the air.

Helping Your Liver

Your liver is the organ chiefly responsible for removing toxins from your body. The process is a complicated one, so I won't go into it in depth here. What you need to know is that it naturally produces a lot of free radicals in the process. Ordinarily, those free radicals are quickly quenched by glutathione, the most abundant antioxidant enzyme in your body. When your liver is busy with extra detoxification, it needs extra glutathione—glutathione that you might not be able to make quickly enough or in large enough quantities. If you can't produce enough glutathione, the free radicals can get the upper hand in your liver and elsewhere, with serious long-term consequences. As I explained earlier, the best way to make sure your levels of glutathione and other antioxidant enzymes stay high is to take in plenty of the vitanutrients that your body needs to manufacture them, such as N-acetyl-cysteine, lipoic acid, and selenium, as well as supplements of glutathione itself. Other vitanutrients equally valuable for supporting your liver include vitamin C, vitamin E, and zinc. The zinc is particularly important for thwarting the activation of carcinogens (cancer-causing substances) as your liver detoxifies them. Lipoic acid and the herb milk thistle are among the vitanutrients best documented to improve liver function.

You also need to support your liver through diet so that it functions at the optimal level and isn't overstrained. This is another area where the low-carbohydrate, high-protein diet pays off. High-quality protein, such as red meat, poultry, seafood, and eggs, enhances detoxification by providing more of the amino acids, especially cysteine, that you need to make glutathione. Your liver needs protein, as well as cholesterol, to manufacture bile, which is essential for absorbing fat-soluble nutrients.

Sugar in any form inhibits the production of the enzymes you need as part of the detoxification process. This will weaken liver function. To strengthen your production of detoxifying enzymes, include lots of cruciferous vegetables in your diet. These members of the cabbage family, including broccoli, kale, and brussels sprouts, are very high in a substance called sulforaphane, which is vital for your liver's ability to convert toxins into nontoxic wastes that can then be removed from your body. And don't forget to drink plenty of pure water every day—at least two quarts (64 ounces, or eight 8-ounce glasses). The water flushes toxins through your system quickly and minimizes their chances to do damage.

Getting the Lead Out

Mercury and lead are two of the most common toxins that can accumulate in your body. Anyone over the age of fifty in America today is quite likely to have accumulated a toxic load of these heavy metals. Not surprisingly, that load can lead to some very serious health problems.

While today's strict regulations have reduced your exposure to lead and mercury to far less than it once was, it is almost certainly still far too high. Old lead plumbing and lead paint are still around, as is all the soil contaminated by the lead that for decades spewed out of the exhaust pipes of millions of vehicles. Mercury is still a major problem, because it constitutes more than half the metal in the silver amalgam fillings used to fill dental cavities. If you've got silver fillings, small amounts of mercury are continuously leaching into your body. This leads to many forms of chronic illness, and worsens life-threatening conditions such as cancer and heart disease.

Over time, absorbing small amounts of lead can cause anemia, neurological damage, high blood pressure, and cardiovascular disease in adults. Small children with high lead levels have impaired mental development that causes learning disabilities and behavioral problems.

The heavy metal cadmium is a by-product of many industrial processes, including zinc smelting. It can be inhaled from polluted air or ingested in contaminated food and water. If your levels of cadmium are high, you're at risk for lung cancer and kidney disease. Recent research shows that high levels of cadmium are also related to bone loss and fractures in older people, especially women. The cadmium increases your excretion of calcium, which in turn leads to thin, brittle bones that break easily.[3]

The best screening tool for both heavy metal accumulation and for the adequacy of essential metals is hair analysis, an inexpensive test that has been inappropriately maligned by conventional medicine. The mineral content of the hair mimics the mineral levels of the entire body. When the report on the hair analysis comes back, you have a good indication of whether toxic minerals are present in excess and whether important minerals, such as chromium, zinc, manganese, and others, are in short supply and in need of supplementation.

Your body has no mechanisms for removing lead, mercury, cadmium, and other heavy metals. Once they get into your system, they're there to stay—unless you remove them through chelation therapy.

Chelation: The Detoxifying Key

Chelation (key-LAY-shun) is a chemical process that captures metal ions in your bloodstream, including lead, iron, calcium, mercury, copper, and zinc, and binds them to an organic molecule. For all intents and purposes, the metal ion is handcuffed to the molecule and can't get away. Instead, it is carried harmlessly out of your body through the urine.

The original use of chelation, starting in the 1930s, was as a treatment for lead poisoning. Then as now, the therapy was administered intravenously. A liquid called ethylenediaminetetraacetic acid (EDTA) is slowly dripped into your blood through a thin needle inserted directly into a vein in your arm.

The EDTA binds to the lead and other metals and removes them. It does not chelate mercury very well, however, so when mercury is the problem we use the chelating agent DMPS or an oral chelator, DMSA.

A typical chelation treatment takes about three hours and is completely painless (after the initial needle stick to insert the IV). To reduce a toxic load of lead or cadmium, you'd probably need to have a total of four to eight sessions. (Your doctor knows when you've had sufficient EDTA; the urine collected after a treatment no longer contains much of the heavy metals.) You'd also need to take zinc and magnesium supplements to replenish the valuable minerals removed by the EDTA. I also prescribe supplements of the complete B complex, with a little extra B_6.

I find that chelation therapy works wonderfully well for many of my patients with elevated heavy metal levels. After the full course of treatments, when their levels drop below detectable amounts, they feel much better.

Although chelation therapy for low-level lead exposure has long been a mainstay of complementary medicine, it is very slowly starting to gain acceptance by the mainstream. A recent study of thirty-two kidney patients, for instance, showed that long-term exposure to low levels of environmental lead has an effect on kidney function—all of them showed mildly elevated blood levels of lead. In the study, the patients were divided into two groups. One group received IV chelation therapy; the other did not. The researchers reported that chelation slowed the progression of renal insufficiency (kidney failure) and actually improved the patients' kidney function by an average of 8.5 percent.[4]

Be skeptical of the oral chelation products that are peddled by some promoters as being just as good as IV chelation for removing toxins from the body. Oral chelation may indeed offer some help for reasons other than their chelating properties, but it simply is not as effective as IV chelation. It is correct to use the term "oral chelation" only for substances that significantly increase the urinary output of heavy metals.

Chelation: Bypassing Bypass Surgery

Overall, chelation therapy is a valuable part of your age-defying program. By removing accumulated heavy metals from your body, you not only remove their harmful effects but also reduce the amount of free radicals they produce. At the Atkins Center, however, we get our most spectacular chelation results in patients with heart disease. We have treated thousands of patients whose conventional doctors warned them that only an immediate angioplasty or heart bypass surgery would save their lives. These patients come to us desperately seeking an alternative to these dangerous procedures, knowing that in fact many bypass patients get worse, not better, after the surgery. They find the alternative they need in chelation therapy—and they also save thousands of dollars. Chelation is far less expensive, and of course far safer, than open-heart surgery or angioplasty.

How exactly does chelation help heart disease? In several different ways. Unlike bypass surgery or angioplasty, which treat just a few of the thousands of arteries in your body, chelation therapy simultaneously increases blood flow in all your major blood vessels, including the ones that nourish your heart, kidneys, brain, and other organs. This happens in part because the EDTA removes some of the calcium found in artery-clogging plaque, which can reduce or sometimes even eliminate the plaque. Even though chelation itself does not reduce or remove plaque, chelation, by removing some calcium from it, allows the plaque to convert to a reversible chemical reaction, in contrast to calcification, which is chemically irreversible. The theory behind the success is that your body's natural enzymes can remove plaque thus rendered soluble.

Chelation also lowers the level of calcium in your blood. This in turn stimulates your body to release parathyroid hormone, which stimulates your body to remove calcium from where it doesn't belong (like in your arteries) and put it where it does (like in your bones). In this way, EDTA causes a modest recalcification of osteoporotic bones.[5]

For heart patients, one of the most valuable benefits of EDTA is the way it stimulates the enlargement of small blood vessels near blocked arteries. These small vessels create collateral circulation around the blockage—your body's own natural bypass. By removing lead, cadmium, and other accumulated heavy metals, chelation removes another cause of heart damage. EDTA is also a powerful antioxidant that can help reduce LDL cholesterol oxidation.[6] Also very helpful for heart patients is EDTA's anticoagulant qualities, which reduce platelet "stickiness" and help prevent the blood clots that can cause a heart attack.[7]

Now that you understand the benefits of chelation therapy, you may be puzzled by the fact that most insurance companies and Medicare refuse to pay for it. These organizations will cheerfully pay $50,000 for you to have bypass surgery, but they won't give you a penny toward the few thousand a complete course of chelation therapy costs.

Conventional physicians often scoff at chelation. Some have even tried to ban it as a treatment. The issue regularly comes up before state medical regulatory boards, but despite what your doctor may tell you, chelation is readily available and perfectly legal just about everywhere in the United States. To find a trained physician who can help you with chelation, check with the American College for Advancement in Medicine

(ACAM) by calling (800) 532–3688 or checking their Web site at www.acam.org.

Mercury Detoxification

Mercury is a highly toxic heavy metal that is extremely dangerous to your health. Mercury exposure is a significant cause of diseases such as multiple sclerosis, cancer, autoimmune disorders, yeast overgrowth, chronic fatigue syndrome, and dozens more. We've all been exposed to considerable amounts of mercury over our lifetime. It's used in many industrial processes and in a wide variety of common chemicals. At one time it was even used in interior housepaint as a way to prevent mildew—a use that was banned several decades ago. There's a very good chance that you are being slowly poisoned by mercury. How? As I hope you realize, it is from the silver amalgam fillings in your teeth.

Detoxification and Dentistry

Although the dental establishment steadfastly denies it, this common material, widely used as an inexpensive method to fill the holes in your teeth left by cavities and root canal procedures, consists of only about 35 percent silver. Half the amalgam is mercury; the rest is a mixture of other metals, including tin, zinc, and copper.

According to the World Health Organization, just one silver amalgam filling in your mouth can release three to seventeen micrograms of mercury a day.[8] Every time you brush your teeth or chew on something, your fillings are releasing tiny amounts of mercury into your body. This is especially true of old fillings, which can corrode over time and release even more mercury.

In Germany, mercury amalgam fillings have been banned since 1992. Here in the United States we are far less enlightened, although some holistic dentists are aware of the issue and refuse to use silver amalgam. Instead, they use polymer ceramic composites. This material is very hard and durable and contains no metals. It's also much more natural looking than silver amalgam. Ceramic fillings are more expensive than standard amalgam fillings. (If you have dental insurance, you'll find that your insurer almost certainly won't pay for the extra cost.)

I urge you to replace all your silver amalgam fillings with ceramic fillings and pay every penny of the cost yourself if necessary. The long-term expense of chronic illness and a shortened life span from the effects of mercury will cost you far more. You may have to search a bit to find a dentist willing to remove your amalgam fillings if you are doing so without a referral from a consultant. If there are no 'diagnosed' medical reasons for their removal you will probably meet with resistance from most dentists.

Sometimes a tooth is so decayed or damaged that the root is affected. To solve the problem, dentists have traditionally done root canal surgery to remove the infected area. There's a big problem with this common procedure— it can leave a residual bacterial infection at the base of the tooth. Toxins from the infection seep into your body and can stimulate chronic degenerative diseases, especially autoimmune disorders. Many of our multiple sclerosis patients at the Atkins Center tell us that their symptoms began soon after they had root canal work involving both infection and silver amalgam fillings. I, along with many other complementary physicians who treat MS, feel that this strong correlation is no coincidence. As part of our treatment protocols for MS, we recommend removing all teeth with root canals and replacing all silver amalgam fillings.

Today's dentists are as dedicated to saving a tooth as physicians are to saving a life. I may be partial to my own profession, but I think saving a life is somehow more important. Having a root canal could jeopardize your health and shorten your life. If possible, take steps to avoid this sort of dental surgery. Good dental hygiene will help you avoid the problem. As a last-resort alternative to a root canal, you may have to have the affected tooth removed instead. Likewise, if you have a degenerative disease such as chronic fatigue syndrome, removing teeth with root canals and replacing all silver amalgam fillings could help restore your health by removing a source of infection and a source of harmful mercury.

Mercury and Your Heart

Cardiologists such as myself, who are aware of environmental toxins, have long known that people with high mercury levels are more likely to have heart failure. This has been confirmed by many studies. The most recent one looked at patients with idiopathic dilated cardiomyopathy, or heart failure with no known cause, and saw that they have extremely high levels of trace elements, particularly mercury and antimony. The levels are astonishing: compared to patients with heart ailments due to a known cause, the heart failure patients had mercury levels that were an astonishing twenty-two thousand times higher.[9]

Heart patients at the Atkins Center are routinely tested for their mercury levels. Just as routinely, we find that the levels are high and must be brought down with chelation therapy.

The only way to remove the accumulated mercury from your system is to take a course of oral chelation therapy. The chelating agent we use is the prescription drug DMSA. Most patients need to take one 500-mg capsule a day for three to eight days. The course ends when a urine sample shows no significant excretion of mercury during the six hours after taking the DMSA capsule.

Now that you've learned about detoxifying your body, as well as some other important age-defying techniques, there's something else you can do to turn your body into an age-defying machine: Exercise!

17

Exercise!

There's one piece of advice I give to virtually every one of my patients, no matter how old: exercise. There's not a one of them who doesn't benefit from exercising regularly to the maximum they can. That doesn't necessarily mean all my patients turn into marathon runners and weekend warriors. What it does mean is that they look better, feel better, and stay healthier. Mentally and physically, they're stronger and more resilient.

Exercise for a Healthy Heart

Without exercise, you'll still benefit from the advice in this book, but with it you'll benefit even more. If you doubt me, just consider the results of a recent review study that looked at dozens of studies on the impact of physical activity on cardiovascular health. Without question, the researchers concluded, regular physical activity provides a wide range of heart-healthy benefits, including lower blood pressure, a drop in cholesterol levels, and a lower risk of dangerous blood clots. The activity doesn't have to be particularly strenuous or prolonged to be effective. Just walking once around the block each day is enough to provide some benefit.[1] Walking more would be better, of course. How much better? According to a recent study of older men in Hawaii, your risk of coronary heart disease decreases 15 percent for every half mile of walking per day.[2]

Earlier studies showed that of all the factors most likely to lead to heart disease, inactivity is at the top of the list, far above all the usual indicators such as high cholesterol.[3] Need I say more? Yes, because exercise does far more for you than just protecting your heart.

The Benefits of Exercise

To defy age, it is crucial to keep your blood sugar levels steady and under control. Exercise is just as important as diet for accomplishing this goal. At the Atkins Center we know how well the combination of exercise and diet works—we've helped thousands of patients with impaired glucose tolerance reverse the process and prolong their lives. Our success is based on the numerous studies—so many that I won't go into them all here—that prove that exercise can prevent, slow, or reverse reduced glucose tolerance and insulin sensitivity as you age and even reverse diabetes if you already have it.

Numerous other studies prove the converse: that not exercising means you're more likely to develop impaired glucose tolerance or diabetes, even if you're not overweight (although being overweight is certainly a contributing factor). A recent study proves this point very powerfully. In this study, more than 8,600 men over age thirty were tracked over a six-year period. Over that time, 149 men in the study developed diabetes. Not very surprisingly, at least to me, the cases were almost entirely among the men who were the least active. Inactive men had nearly four times the risk of developing diabetes compared with physically active men.[4]

Having an active lifestyle is also linked with a reduced risk of cancer, as has been demonstrated in regard to colon cancer in men and breast cancer in women.[5]

For those of you who need to lose weight, regular exercise will help speed the process along. I particularly recommend it for people who have a high metabolic resistance to weight loss. Even though walking a mile burns only a hundred calories, a long-term exercise program often proves to be the essential factor that tips the balance in hard-core unable-to-lose-on-a-strict-diet people. Those of you whose weight loss is simply pla-teauing will find that exercise will also get you over the logjam more quickly. Best of all, the experience of seeing your fat turn into muscle, and of knowing that you're capable of many more physical achievements, is such a mood lifter that your all-around well-being will reach new heights.

The Bigger Picture

Exercise is the key factor in preventing disability as you age. It's also a key factor in overall longevity. Let's look at some statistics to prove my point.

Overall, a sixty-five-year-old man with no disabilities in the United States today has only a 26 percent chance of living to age eighty and remaining disability free. For a woman, the probability of living to age eighty-five and remaining disability free is only 18 percent. What do the minority who are disability free do to get and stay that way? They exercise. People who exercise regularly have a lower risk of becoming disabled later in life than those who don't exercise. And the people with the highest level of physical activity are nearly twice as likely to be disability free as the most sedentary.[6]

What the numbers show most starkly is that disability is not an inevitable part of aging. It can easily be defied by moderate physical activity, starting now.

Physical activity can also extend your life expectancy. Among nonsmokers at age sixty-five, moderate physical activity is associated with 14.4 years of continuing life expectancy in men and 16.2 years in women. In other words, a man who exercises moderately and doesn't smoke is likely to live to be just over seventy-nine years old. That's a gain of seven years over the average life expectancy of seventy-two years for a man.

The benefits of physical activity hold true even for smokers. Male smokers who exercise moderately gain 10.5 years of extra life expectancy; women gain 12.6 years.[7] What better reason could there be to start your age-defying exercise program today?

Exercising Your Options

Despite the perfectly obvious benefits of exercising, some 30 percent of the American population doesn't exercise at all. These couch potatoes have opted, whether they realize it or not, for a shortened life span marred at the end by years of expensive, painful disability. What will you opt for? Will you choose to exercise and defy age, or remain inactive and court disability and premature death? It's a simple choice, really, and yet many of my patients have trouble making the commitment to exercise. I've heard every excuse in the book, and although I'm certainly guilty of some of them myself, none of them are valid.

Patients tell me all the time that they just don't have time to exercise. Nonsense! If the average American can find time to watch six hours of television a day, he or she can find time for half an hour of exercise. If you can't bear to miss a minute of TV time, ride an exercise bike or do stretching exercises and calisthenics while you watch.

Another big excuse I hear is being too old to exercise. This is just as nonsensical as the lack of time excuse. It's never too late to start an exercise program. In one study, a group of frail, nonagenarian men living in a nursing home did weight training! In just eight weeks they showed remarkable increases in muscle strength of up to 175 percent. More important, their walking speed and coordination improved by nearly 50 percent, making them much less likely to have a fall.[8] Several other studies since then have shown similar results, improving walking speed and overall strength and improving measures of physical disability.[9]

"Exercise is so boring," some of my patients say. "Maybe so," is my reply, "but it's a lot less boring than living in a nursing home." Find a form of exercise you enjoy and do it regularly. Golf, tennis, walking, hiking, biking, dancing, swimming—all will roll back the clock. And even constructive activities such as gardening, housework, home repairs, and the like can be done in such a way that they are meaningful sources of exercise.

Of all the excuses I hear, the least convincing is that you are too out of shape to exercise. That's exactly what we're going to remedy!

Walking to Better Health

The form of exercise I recommend most, especially if you're just starting an exercise program, is walking. If you start by simply taking a short walk every day, or even every other day, you will notice dramatic improvements in a very short time.

It matters little how far or how fast you go or how old you are. In a recent study from Japan, for example, middle-age men who walked just ten to twenty minutes a day, five days a week, reduced their risk of hypertension by 12 percent and lost weight.[10]

A recent study, even more to the point, followed nearly three thousand American men age seventy-one to ninety-three for four years. During that time, 109 of the men were diagnosed with coronary artery disease. What's interesting is the breakdown. The men who walked one and a half miles a day or more had a 2.5 percent risk of heart disease. The men who walked less than a quarter of a mile a day had double the risk, or a 5 percent chance of heart disease.[11] In other words, by spending half an hour taking a relaxing walk, these older men cut their risk of heart disease in half, to say nothing of the other benefits they reaped.

The benefits of walking might be even more dramatic for women. According to a recent study of participants in the ongoing Nurses' Health Study, fully one-third of heart attacks in women of any age could be prevented by three hours of brisk walking (twenty minutes per mile) spread over a week. A woman who walks briskly for five or more hours a week cuts her heart attack risk in half. The benefit applies to all women, even sedentary ones who take up walking later in life. There's no real reason to think what works for women won't also work for men.[12]

What other benefits does walking give you? Well, aside from the health advantages I've already discussed for any sort of exercise, walking seems to improve your mental fitness. In particular, a recent study shows that walking improves what are known as the executive control functions—your ability to plan, coordinate, and focus on information. The study compared two groups of previously sedentary older adults. One group walked for forty-five minutes three times a week. The other group did stretching and toning exercises for an hour three times a week. When the two groups were given a battery of psychological tests after six months, the walkers did much better. What seems to have made the difference is the increased flow of blood to the brain that came with walking.[13]

Walking has several other benefits to commend it to you. It is a weight-bearing form of exercise, which is an important aspect of preventing or slowing osteoporosis. Walking is far gentler on your body than jogging or running and is unlikely to injure you. Unlike more strenuous forms of exercise, walking does not have a negative effect on your immune system. Jogging for just half an hour every day can significantly reduce the number of immune cells in your blood, but walking half an hour a day will have at the least no effect on your immunity and may well give it a boost.[14]

One of the best things about walking is that it requires no special equipment beyond a comfortable pair of sneakers or shoes. You also don't need any special training—you've been walking all your life. And it's free—no gym fees, no fancy equipment, no instructors.

Your age-defying goal is to take a brisk half-hour walk at least three times a week, and preferably every day. The time you spend walking is more important than the distance you cover. If you haven't walked more than a couple of blocks in years, start slowly by walking as quickly as is comfortable for just ten minutes. Gradually work up to half an hour, keeping the pace at whatever is comfortable for you. You'll be amazed at how quickly you get up to half an hour and at how much better you feel, both physically and mentally. In fact, you may feel so good that you decide to walk longer or more frequently, which in turn will make you feel even better.

As you walk, be aware of your posture. We all have a natural tendency as we get older to stoop forward a bit, a tendency that can be quite pronounced in the elderly. You need to counteract the tendency before it happens. The farther forward you stoop, the more likely you are to have a fall that could break a bone.

Check your posture by standing naturally up against a wall and seeing how much of you touches it. If the back of your head doesn't touch the wall, you'll need to take some corrective steps. Try to stand so that your head *does* touch the wall. You'll find that it works better if you pull your abdomen in, tilt your hips forward, and try to elevate your chest away from your pelvis. This is the very posture you should strive for when walking.

As you walk, hold your chin up, along with the back of your head. Once your head is balanced more naturally over your shoulders, the rest of your posture will straighten up as well. By constantly reminding yourself to keep your head back, you'll overcome your forward stoop.

When More Is Less

If mild exercise is good and moderate exercise is better, does that make heavy exercise the best? Precisely the opposite. Aside from increasing the chances of an injury, heavy exercise makes you produce an overabundance of free radicals, has a detrimental effect on your immune system, and makes you release more of the damaging stress hormone cortisol. That's why I don't recommend running or jogging as exercise. Swimming, walking, yoga, and other slower, gentler activities—even housework—when done regularly, have just as beneficial an effect on your body without all the extra wear and tear.

If you have arthritis or some other condition that impairs

your mobility, I still recommend walking as much as you can. I also recommend water exercises under the supervision of a trained physical or exercise therapist. Many local Ys and community pools offer inexpensive water exercise classes.

By the way, anyone who thinks he or she is achieving immortality the Ornish way by running forty miles a week and eating a very low-fat diet is in for a surprise. A recent study showed that when high-mileage runners ate a diet in which only 17 percent of the calories came from fat, their levels of infection-fighting white blood cells and cytokines plummeted, while their levels of cortisol and inflammation-producing prostaglandins increased. When the runners went to a high-fat diet with 41 percent of the calories from fat, their levels returned to normal—and their level of natural killer cells, which attack viruses and tumor cells, doubled.[15] Scientific studies don't usually discuss how the subjects actually feel, but I'm sure in this case that the subjects felt a lot better in general when they were eating the high-fat diet. I'm also sure they were a lot less likely to get sick with the sort of minor ailments, like colds and infections, that dog many serious athletes who follow fat-restricted diets.

Stretching the Truth

As great an age-defier as walking is, it is tied for first place in my mind with another activity that is invaluable and not at all strenuous—stretching.

I don't think I have to remind you that stiffness and progressive inflexibility of the spine and other joints are well-known concomitants of aging. Loosening up these joints by putting the tight muscles around them "on the stretch" is a dramatically effective correction for this problem.

There are more than a hundred different stretching exercises that can benefit your different muscle groups. It's not within the scope of this book to provide the details—you can get them from the many good books on the topic or from an exercise instructor at your local Y or health club. I merely want to point out that stretches provide an invaluable protection against the musculoskeletal problems associated with advancing years.

Aerobics and Weight Training

The next vital concept to work toward is adopting a program of aerobic exercise. The object is to create a need for a comfortable increase in your body's oxygen requirements and pulse rate and keep it constant for a meaningful time. For many of you, half an hour of brisk walking will do it; for others, it will take more. If more exercise is required, swimming, jogging, bicycling, aerobics classes, and the like are all appropriate, providing they are not so vigorous that they stress your immune reserves or lead to injury.

The third valuable exercise possibility is resistance training, also known as weight training. Resistance training is done primarily to strengthen muscles. It can also be moderately aerobic, especially when done with lighter weights. As mentioned earlier, research has shown that even frail elderly people can benefit from weight training. To avoid injury when you're first getting started with weights, I suggest working with a certified trainer to learn the basics.

Getting Started

If you're over age forty-five, before you undertake any exercise program more strenuous than brisk walking, see your doctor and get yourself examined for any cardiovascular problems.

To avoid injuries, always do some stretching and limbering exercises before you get into the more active part of your exercise routine. If you're just beginning an exercise program, start slowly. Forget the saying, "No pain, no gain." At first, do a little bit *less* than you think you can, not a little bit more. Gradually build up to a level that leaves you feeling energized and refreshed, not exhausted and sore. Over the first few weeks, you'll be amazed at how quickly you get into better shape. After that, your progress may be a bit slower. Set realistic goals for yourself and remember that you're not training for the Olympics.

When you exercise, there should be a normal elevation of your pulse rate. If you feel dizzy, have chest pains, or feel very short of breath, STOP. Check things out with your physician before you exercise to that level again. Avoid exercising outdoors in extremely hot or cold weather. When the weather is against you, you can walk at your local shopping mall or on a treadmill.

Regular exercise is habit-forming, if not downright addictive. You'll find that it easily becomes a routine and very pleasant part of your life. Now that you're on the road to a sound body, let's look at lifelong ways to keep a sound mind in that body.

18

Boost Your Brain Power

Whenever patients ask me about one of their aging relatives, I usually start by asking, "What do you think of his or her short-term memory?" That symptom may well be the most consistent shortcoming found in people who are suffering the effects of aging as we know it.

Medically speaking, the problem goes by the name age-related memory loss. That term would make you think that some loss of the ability to recall the events of the previous day or the names of familiar people is an unavoidable expectation as you get older. It is not.

There are too many nutrients that seem to make a difference in maintaining, or even improving, not only your memory but all aspects of your brain power for memory loss to be inevitable. It's just a matter of deciding which of these safe and effective nutrients are the best for you.

Protecting Your Brain

Everything you do to protect your body from aging applies even more to your brain. That's because your brain is much more vulnerable than the rest of your body to the effects of free radicals and reduced blood flow. Why is your brain so unprotected?

Your brain consists of trillions of nerve cells, or neurons, all packed very closely together into an organ that weighs only about three pounds. All those cells communicate with one another and with the rest of your body through complex chemical messengers called neurotransmitters.

Even though your brain takes up only about 2 percent of your body mass, it demands more than 25 percent of your body's basic fuels, glucose or ketones, to run at peak efficiency.

The best studied is glucose (the fuel used on a balanced diet), so I'll describe how the brain uses it. Unlike many other substances in your bloodstream, glucose passes easily through the blood-brain barrier. And unlike the cells everywhere else in your body, brain cells don't need insulin to carry the glucose into them. Brain cells are very sensitive to glucose, however—too little or too much causes damage or death. If your brain cells don't need insulin, how does your body control how much glucose gets in? Through a very complex system of hormones and feedback loops, all designed to keep your blood glucose stable on the other side of the blood-brain barrier. In other words, if your body's blood sugar stays stable, your brain's will as well. The reverse is also true. If your body's blood sugar zooms up and down, or stays consistently too high, the instability will take a toll on your brain as well as the rest of your body.

Too much glucose entering your brain has exactly the same effect as too much glucose anywhere else in your body. It causes AGEs (advanced glycosylation end-products), atherosclerosis, reduced oxygen flow, and, of course, major free radical damage. We know that AGEs contribute to the plaques made of a type of protein called beta amyloid that are found in the brains of Alzheimer's patients.[1]

What if your brain doesn't get enough glucose? Then the hormonal feedback loop first calls on glucagon, the hormone that counterbalances insulin, to raise your glucose level. If that doesn't work—and in people with unstable blood sugar it doesn't—then the next step is to call on cortisol, the stress hormone. Your body is designed to use cortisol only when it's suddenly urgent to raise your blood sugar, like when you're in a threatening situation. If unstable blood sugar frequently forces your body to fall back on cortisol, the long-term effects on your brain are very bad. To be blunt, cortisol kills brain cells. To be specific, it kills brain cells in your hippocampus, the part of your brain that tells the rest of your brain to start the hormonal cascades. Your hippocampus is also involved in the process that turns short-term memory into long-term memory. It's easy to see that too much cortisol, and the damage it causes to your hippocampus cells, is something you really don't need.

A third blood-sugar-elevating hormone, and one whose effects are very easy to notice, is adrenaline. The adrenalinelike neurotransmitters create an anxiety/fear emotional response characterized by rapid heartbeat, dry mouth, and sweaty palms, which explains why panic attacks and bouts of heart rhythm irregularities are triggered by falling blood sugar. Even worse, such physical and emotional stress will cause further cortisol elevations. Clearly, maintaining stable blood sugar is essential for protecting your brain.

Your brain is also a glutton for oxygen. More than 20 percent of the oxygen in your blood goes to your brain. If the blood vessels that carry blood to and from your brain become stiff or partially blocked, oxygen flow to your brain is reduced, along with the flow of everything else your brain needs. Poor cerebral circulation causes slow, steady loss of brain function: poor memory, confusion, inability to concentrate, fatigue, depression, anxiety. It also sharply increases your chance of a major stroke.

When the overall blood flow to your brain is reduced, the damage caused by lack of oxygen, glucose, and antioxidants lets free radicals get the upper hand. Free radical damage anywhere in your body is bad. In your brain, it can be devastating. Over the long term, anything that causes free radical damage reduces brain function. Conversely, over the long term, anything that reduces free radical damage preserves brain function.

How to Help Your Brain

You may have heard the folk wisdom that you lose a hundred thousand brain cells every day as you age. It is true that some of your neurons naturally die off as you get older, but in healthy aging, neuron loss is actually fairly minimal—and it happens only in some areas of the brain. It's also not true that you never grow any new neurons. In fact, even elderly people create hundreds of new neurons every day. When a neuron does die, other neurons in the area pick up the slack and create new connections with other brain cells. Just as an experienced older tennis player who can't run as fast as he used to can still win a match against a younger, faster, but less-experienced player, so does your brain compensate for the loss of neurons.

The process works a lot better, of course, if you give your brain a little help. As with your body, that help should consist of diet and exercise. By diet I mean the same low-carbohydrate, high-antioxidant, high-fat diet that helps the rest of your body. This is one of the few times I will emphasize the high-fat part of the diet. That's because certain fats are extremely important for your brain. Without enough essential fatty acids—fats you must get from your food—your brain just won't work right (check back to Chapter 14 for more on essential fatty acids).

The low-fat diet the medical establishment insists is good for you stands a better chance of eventually slowing your brain than helping to keep it going strong. New studies support this, such as one showing that the typical high-fat Western diet is linked to a lower risk of poststroke dementia. The study looked at a group of older Japanese-American men who had had strokes. The men who preferred a Western-style diet to the traditional low-fat Japanese diet were about half as likely to develop stroke-related dementia (an aftermath of stroke where the brain does not fully recover). The researchers believe that the high fat intake of the Western diet acts as a stabilizer to the small arteries in the brain.[2]

Your brain needs exercise just as the rest of your body does. Several studies show, for instance, that people with higher levels of education are less likely to develop Alzheimer's disease as they age.[3] The reason may well be that these people continue to stay mentally active through their work and through their leisure. You don't need a Ph.D. to read, listen to music, do crossword puzzles, or enjoy a hobby or take up a new one. Staying engaged and active in your community and social life also helps keep your mind sharp. Socializing with family and friends and participating in group activities have been shown to reduce stress levels—and therefore brain-damaging cortisol levels.[4] Anything that keeps your brain engaged will do a lot to keep it healthy.

Brain Vitanutrients

Every few months, a new patient comes to the Atkins Center complaining of forgetfulness. Suddenly, he or she just can't remember minor things, like the name of the boss's wife, that used to come easily to mind. After doing some simple memory tests and a quick exam, I'm almost always able to give these patients good news. All they're experiencing is normal, age-related changes in their short-term memory. If you're over forty-five, you're likely to be experiencing the same thing. Do you now have to spend the rest of your life forgetting phone numbers? No. You're fortunate to live in a time when research into brain vitanutrients is moving along very rapidly. The vitanutrients I'll discuss in this chapter are excellent for maintaining and improving total mental function, including short-term memory.

Ginkgo Biloba

I've already discussed ginkgo biloba as an excellent antioxidant vitanutrient earlier in the book. Here I'll focus on the use of ginkgo to maintain and improve your mental acuity, an area where I consider ginkgo to be the top nutrient of them all.

We know from more than forty research studies that the active ingredients in ginkgo biloba are very effective for increasing blood flow to the brain. Better blood flow means better memory and more alertness overall. Numerous studies have shown that in cases of cerebral insufficiency (poor blood flow to the brain), ginkgo is a valuable and extremely safe treatment. By restoring a more normal blood flow to the brain, ginkgo reduces or even eliminates memory loss, confusion, disorientation, and agitation. Of course, better blood flow also means less likelihood of a stroke. Ginkgo reduces your chances of a stroke in another way, by making your platelets less sticky and therefore less likely to clot and block blood flow to your brain.

Ginkgo can help slow down and perhaps stop or even reverse some of the brain damage from Alzheimer's disease (AD).[5] Ginkgo is an approved treatment for AD in Germany and some other countries. Several recent studies in the United States have shown that taking ginkgo can stabilize and even improve Alzheimer's-type dementia for up to a year. In the studies, the patients taking ginkgo had stable or improved cognitive function. They did as well as other patients taking more expensive prescription drugs, without the side effects, and they did markedly better than patients who took only a placebo.[6]

Always choose a ginkgo supplement in tablet form that has been standardized to 24 percent ginkgo flavonoids and 6 percent terpenes. For adults over forty, I recommend taking at least 60 mg (the amount in one tablet) three times a day, for a total of 180 mg. For adults over sixty, or if you're experiencing short-term memory loss, increase the dose to two or even three 60 mg tablets at a time, up to three times a day, for a total of 240 to 360 mg. Even doses much larger than this are perfectly safe. Ginkgo has no known toxicity or side effects, and it has no known interactions with other drugs or nutrients.

When you take ginkgo biloba to improve general alertness and mental acuity, the effect is felt almost immediately. Ginkgo isn't a stimulant, though, and it won't keep you up at night or make you jittery.

For improving short-term memory (the reason I recommend ginkgo most), you'll need to take ginkgo for at least a couple of weeks before you start noticing a change for the better. It happens gradually, but almost all of my patients experience significant short-term memory improvement within three months.

Phosphatidyl Serine (PS)

If there was a safe, inexpensive dietary supplement that could turn back a decade's worth of mental decline, would you take it? I bet you would. Well, there is such a supplement—it's called phosphatidyl serine (PS). This one is providing especially exciting results, and I find it every bit as effective as—and complementary to—ginkgo.

Phosphatidyl serine is a naturally occurring phospholipid found in the fatty membranes of all your cells. (Phospholipids are large fatty molecules that are the universal building blocks for all the cell membranes in your body.) The membranes of your brain cells are particularly rich in PS, because PS plays an important role both in releasing neurotransmitters and increasing the number of neurotransmitter receptor sites on each cell. That gives your brain more circuits with which to communicate. As you age, though, your brain cells start to make less and less PS, to the point where eventually your cognitive ability is impaired. The deterioration will happen faster if you're also low on the building blocks for manufacturing PS in your body, including folic acid, vitamin B_{12}, and essential fatty acids, particularly the omega-3 oils.

Taken as a supplement, PS can be little short of miraculous as a way to boost your memory, improve your concentration, and brighten your mood. It's particularly helpful for improving short-term memory in older adults, as shown by a study of 149 people age fifty or older with "normal" age-related memory loss. Some of the study participants took 100 mg of PS three times a day for twelve weeks; the rest took a placebo. At the end of the experiment, the PS group showed a 15 percent improvement in learning and memory tasks. The most improvement came from the people who were most impaired entering the study. Interestingly, the benefits continued for up to four weeks after the participants stopped taking PS.[7]

PS can also help prevent damage to the brain and other organs caused by excessive cortisol production. In a recent well-designed study of people who exercised intensely, PS kept cortisol levels from rising sharply.[8] Even if you don't exercise a lot, anything that keeps your brain from being bombarded by cortisol will help preserve your cognitive function.

Phosphatidyl serine is found naturally in very small amounts in many common foods. Even lecithin, which contains other phospholipids such as phosphatidyl choline, doesn't have enough PS to raise your body levels in any significant way. To get the amounts you need to improve cognition, you will simply have to take supplements of PS. Until recently, that was a somewhat chancy proposition, because PS supplements were made from cow brains and carried a slight risk of viral infection. Today, however, PS supplements are made from soybeans and are quite safe to take. I recommend taking anywhere from 100 to 300 mg a day, preferably just before breakfast and lunch. The effects of supplemental PS continue for up to four weeks after you stop taking it. This allows you, if you are concerned about the cost of PS (at the present writing, 100 mg cost about $1), to taper the dosage once you have achieved a maximum apparent benefit. You can then cut back to perhaps 60 to 100 mg without losing the brain-enhancing effect.

Because PS is a fat, it's vulnerable to free radical damage as it circulates in your body on its way to your brain. By following the entire age-defying protocol, which includes lots of antioxidant nutrients, you should have no trouble protecting the investment you're making in mental maintenance.

Choline

Choline, a member of the B vitamin family, is needed to make the phospholipid phosphatidyl choline (lecithin); it's also needed to make the neurotransmitter acetylcholine.

Choline has recently gotten a reputation as a useful overall memory booster. A choline supplement called DMAE (2-

dimethylaminoethanol, also sometimes called deaner) is available, and it may be the best version of choline to use. In animal studies, DMAE has been shown to improve memory and learning capacity, perhaps by raising phosphatidyl choline levels in the animals' brains. Even though there are few studies showing that it works in humans, several of my patients insist that DMAE has helped their brain function. But please don't overlook the best dietary source of phosphatidyl choline: egg yolks.

Docosahexaenoic Acid (DHA)

Another major building block for brain cell membranes is docosahexaenoic acid, better known as DHA. We know that infants and young children need to get plenty of DHA from their food for their rapidly growing brains to develop fully. Today there's increasing evidence to show that DHA is essential for mental functioning in all stages of life, from infancy to old age. DHA is actually an omega-3 fatty acid that you get from your food. Like EPA, another important omega-3 fatty acid, it's found primarily in cold-water fish such as salmon and cod. If chickens are fed well, their egg yolks can be a great source of DHA. Organic eggs are generally measureably higher in DHA than factory-farm eggs. Also, if you take EPA supplements, you get a fair amount of DHA as well. You could also try the newer DHA capsules that are very low in EPA.

We have just begun to use higher doses of DHA at the Atkins Center, and we are already hearing some gratifying feedback from patients taking doses in the 1,000- to 3,000-mg range.

Acetyl-l-Carnitine (ALC)

The amino acid carnitine is one of my favorite vitanutrients. I use it extensively to treat heart disease, metabolic resistance to weight loss, and fatigue.

Acetyl-l-carnitine (ALC) is a sort of supercarnitine. In many ways it's very similar to carnitine, but its molecular structure makes it easier to absorb than carnitine. It is also much more capable of benefiting your brain. It can improve memory and alertness, slow the aging of brain cells, and energize your entire nervous system. A number of studies have also shown that ALC can slow the mental decline that comes with Alzheimer's disease and other forms of dementia.[9] ALC isn't just for the elderly, however; it enhances mental performance in everyone, even twenty-somethings.

In general, ALC enhances the ability of your cells to produce energy by transporting fat molecules into the mitochondria, where they can be burned as fuel. While it's there in the mitochondria, ALC also functions as a potent antioxidant that snuffs out free radicals as soon as they're created. In your brain, ALC is a crucial part of the process for creating the neurotransmitter acetylcholine. I've already discussed the value of ALC for counteracting the aging effects of excess cortisol (see Chapter 12).

In your body, natural processes convert carnitine to the acetyl-l form, but only in small amounts. For the most effective ALC supplementation, then, carnitine supplements alone won't do the trick—ALC supplements will be much more effective. If you're a generally healthy person over forty, taking 500 to 1,000 mg of ALC daily will help improve your mental performance. As an added benefit, the ALC supplements will raise your overall carnitine level. One word of caution: ALC invigorates your brain so well that it could keep you from sleeping. Take your ALC supplements in the morning.

Pregnenolone

Back in Chapter 12, I discussed the many uses of the grandmother hormone pregnenolone. Here I'll focus just on how pregnenolone can reverse age-related declines in memory and improve mental performance.

Pregnenolone works by enhancing your ability to transmit impulses from neuron to neuron. The faster and more efficiently the impulses travel, the faster your brain works. Studies with lab animals show that even very small doses of pregnenolone markedly improve their ability to learn and remember.[10] Very similar results have recently been documented in humans. Pregnenolone has been shown to improve memory in older adults as measured by standard memory tests.[11] In my experience, patients who take pregnenolone for other reasons still report feeling sharper and more focused. The ones who take pregnenolone specifically for memory notice definite improvements.

A daily dose of up to 100 mg of pregnenolone should be sufficient to notice an uptick in mental function.

The B Vitamins

The entire B vitamin complex—from thiamin through cobalamin (vitamin B_{12})—is essential for proper brain function. Among other things, you need all the B vitamins in order to make neurotransmitters. If you're low on any one of the B vitamins, you're very likely to be low on the others as well. Even a very mild deficiency of any of the B vitamins can cause cognitive problems such as memory loss, confusion, anxiety, depression, and sleep disorders.

I believe that deficiencies of B vitamins are an often overlooked cause of many cases of so-called senile dementia. The B vitamins in general are difficult to absorb from food. As we get older, our bodies have an even harder time taking them in. Combine that with the fact that many older people don't take in enough calories, and that the calories they do take in often come from foods low in B vitamins, and you practically have a formula for deficiency.

I've discussed the value of all the B vitamins at length in other works.* Here I'll discuss just two of them in detail. The first is the one B vitamin that anyone over age fifty is most likely to be deficient in: cobalamin, also known as vitamin B_{12}. The second is folic acid, the B vitamin that protects not just your heart but also your brain.

Your level of vitamin B_{12} is seriously affected by aging. That's because to absorb B_{12} from your food, your stomach uses not only its usual hydrochloric acid and pepsin but also a special substance called intrinsic factor. As you age, however, you progressively make less and less of all your digestive fluids, including intrinsic factor. If you're over age sixty, there's a 50–50 chance that you're no longer making enough intrinsic factor to absorb all the vitamin B_{12} you need from your food. The result is the slow, insidious development of a B_{12} deficiency, along with symptoms of "senility." A serious B_{12} deficiency shows up easily on a blood test, because it causes a very obvious type of anemia. Mild B_{12} deficiency isn't visible on a blood test, however, and older people who are just on the low end of normal can still show symptoms of deficiency.

In fact, the prevalence of vitamin B_{12} deficiency among older adults is startlingly high. According to a recent study, some 40 percent of the population over age sixty-seven have suboptimal levels, and 12 percent have outright deficiency.[12]

B_{12} deficiency develops slowly, often starting years before anyone would consider you elderly. The damage it causes happens gradually and can't always be reversed. I prefer to see all my patients over age fifty supplement with vitamin B_{12}. Injec-

*Please see *Dr. Atkins' Vita-Nutrient Solution* for details.

tions are the gold standard for administering vitamin B_{12}. The proper dose is 1 cc containing 1 mg of the vitamin, given monthly. Oral forms of B_{12} are subject to the same intrinsic factor shortage that inhibits absorption from food. Oral doses over 1,000 mg do get absorbed, however, so if you want to take an oral form, the dose needs to be at least that large.

Folic Acid

I've already discussed how important folic acid is to the health of your heart. The benefits also apply to your brain, and for the same reason. Folic acid lowers the amount of artery-damaging homocysteine in your blood, which helps prevent not just heart attacks but also strokes and reduced cerebral circulation from hardened arteries in the brain. High homocysteine levels are also related to Alzheimer's disease. People with Alzheimer's tend to have low blood levels of both folic acid and vitamin B_{12} and moderately elevated blood levels of homocysteine. In a recent study, researchers looked at homocysteine levels in two groups of people over age fifty-five—one group that had Alzheimer's disease and one that didn't. The people with the highest level of homocysteine were 4.5 times more likely to have Alzheimer's than those with the lowest level. Similarly, those with the lowest level of folic acid were 3.3 times more likely to have Alzheimer's, while those with the lowest vitamin B_{12} level were 4.3 times more likely to have it.[13]

Even though the FDA has mandated that processed grain foods such as bread, baked goods, and breakfast cereals now contain supplemental folic acid, the official recommended daily intake is only a pitiful 800 mcg. I believe that is far too low to have any positive effect on your health. I suggest that basically healthy people take at least 3 to 8 mg a day—more for those with a family history of heart disease, stroke, or early senility.

Not the SAMe Old Thing

One of the hottest new antiaging supplements today is S-adenosylmethionine, better known as SAMe. At the Atkins Center we have mainly used this natural version of the amino acid methionine as a safe, drug-free treatment for depression and for arthritis, but now there may be another reason to prescribe SAMe. Recent research shows that Alzheimer's patients have very low SAMe levels in their brains. This was something of a surprise to the researchers, because earlier studies had shown that these patients had high levels of SAMe—but in their blood. There still haven't been any studies of whether supplemental SAMe will help slow Alzheimer's disease.[14]

Is SAMe helpful for ordinary brain aging? It's simply too early to tell.

"Smart" Drugs

Because I have a bit of a reputation as an "alternative" doctor, hardly a day goes by without my getting promotional material about some new "smart drug" that's supposed to enhance your brain power and reverse the aging process. I'm familiar with many of these drugs from my contacts with colleagues in Europe, where much of the research in this area goes on. Some of these drugs do indeed have some merit, but I don't prescribe them often, mainly because the vitanutrients I've just described seem to benefit so many of my patients. The drugs' benefits are generally outweighed by their drawbacks, expense, and unavailability. Most of these medications aren't readily available in the United States, even though they're sometimes sold over the counter in Europe.

"Smart drugs" such as deprenyl, hydergine, vinpocetin, piracetam, and others are not do-it-yourself medicine. These are prescription drugs, not dietary supplements, and there are risks to using them. You need to work closely with a physician who is accustomed to using these drugs. Even then, I feel strongly that the same benefits can be achieved more effectively through nutrition, with less trouble and expense and far less risk.

Now it's time to take everything I've discussed up to this point and put it all together into a diet program that will help you stay healthy and active as long as possible. As you'll discover in Part IV, there's nothing mysterious or complex about my age-defying diet. It's easy to understand and easy to follow—and it works.

PART V

Living the
Age-Defying Diet

In this part I detail the heart of this book: how to live the age-defying diet. Here you'll learn the basics of the diet:

■

How to defy conventional wisdom and ignore the "food pyramid."

■

How to select low-carbohydrate, nutrient-dense foods that stabilize your blood sugar and are also rich sources of antioxidants.

■

How to choose the right fats and avoid the dangerous ones.

■

How to tailor the diet to your individual needs and discover the carbohydrate intake level that is best for you.

■

How to decide which supplements you need to take, and in what amounts.

19

Creating Your Age-Defying Diet

I assume there are some of you who are starting to read this book at this point. If you're just joining me, here's what you would have learned already—and if you've read through to this point, here's a useful review of my main points.

- The greatest inhibitor of a full life span is atherosclerosis—vital arteries blocked by plaque.
- Atherosclerosis is a condition of our distorted modern diet, one that has been in existence (except in rare, isolated cases) for less than a century. Further, you now know that atherosclerosis is part and parcel of an insulin disorder—excessive insulin—that develops only among people who consume a diet made up mostly of refined carbohydrates, especially junk carbohydrates such as white flour, sugar, and corn syrup.
- The insulin disorder leads to unhealthful elevations of blood glucose, a characteristic of diabetes and related disorders. Elevations of glucose in turn lead inexorably to premature aging by creating AGEs (advanced glyco-

249

sylation end products), caused when the extra sugar in your system combines with essential body proteins.

- Insulin, the hormone that naturally brings your sugar levels down, is extremely atherogenic (causative of atherosclerosis).

- Logically, then, the best way to avoid the glucose versus insulin dilemma is to follow a low-glycemic diet that is the least able to raise your glucose and insulin levels.

- Because carbohydrates are all, to some extent, glycemic, and because noncarbohydrate foods are barely glycemic at all, simple logic tells you—and my patients have proved over and over again—that a low-carbohydrate diet (also known as a low-glycemic diet) will correct the most prevalent cause of atherosclerosis.

- If you're overweight, a low-carbohydrate diet causes an automatic loss of weight by switching your primary source of energy fuel to stored body fat. If your weight is normal or below normal, however, the low-carbohydrate diet must be modified for you to prevent the production of excess insulin but also maintain your weight.

Put all the above together and you have a pretty clear idea of the first essential point of any age-defying diet: *No matter what your weight, you must reduce the amount of refined carbohydrates in your diet.* And if you do need to lose weight, the low-carbohydrate diet is the best, easiest, safest, and most luxurious way to do it.

Let me be perfectly clear about this: The age-defying diet, like my weight-loss diet, is a low-carbohydrate diet. It is *not* a low-calorie diet—you will never have to go hungry, much less starve yourself, on any diet I suggest.

Now let's move on to the next age-defying step. You've also learned:

- Most aging theorists agree that free radical activity is a primary cause of the symptoms of aging. Nutritional antioxidants play a well-established and well-proven role in preventing aging.
- Antioxidants from food may prove more valuable than the antioxidants given as nutritional supplements. Vegetables and fruits contain significant amounts of antioxidant flavonoids and other beneficial phytochemicals, so many that we haven't begun to identify them all yet. Supplements are often needed to give you an extra antioxidant boost, but drinking green tea and eating plenty of fresh vegetables and low-sugar fruits gives you the best variety of flavonoids.
- There is a wide disparity in nutritional value and glucose content even among foods in the same category. Among fruits, for instance, bananas are little more than unwanted carbohydrates, but blueberries are relatively low in sugar and very high in antioxidants. The *quality* of your food selections assumes paramount importance.

Put all this together, and you've got the second essential point of your age-defying diet: *You need a diet that is high in antioxidants, primarily from fresh vegetables and low-sugar fruits and also from supplements as needed.*

Now let's look at the third and perhaps most important part of your age-defying diet:

- We are all individuals, with different genetic predispositions, different histories, different health problems to overcome, different tastes in food, and different metabolic responses. *Therefore, one diet cannot fit all.*

Before I go into detail about how to create your own age-defying diet, let me make one last point. Diet alone will make a big difference in how you age, but we also need to remember three other crucial components that fend off the symptoms of aging: hormones, brain nutrients, and exercise.

I've discussed all those factors in earlier chapters, so here I'm just reminding you that you need to include them all in your overall age-defying strategy. Used intelligently, under proper medical supervision if necessary, all three components can help slow the aging process and give you better mental and physical health.

Planning Your Age-Defying Diet

Armed with all these facts, what age-defying diet is best for you? That's a good question. There isn't an "Atkins Age-Defying Diet" that works for everybody. But I can do for you what I do for each patient who sees me privately in consultation: *teach you basic dietary principles and help you select an eating program that applies best to you.*

Your personal program will be based on the age-defying principles, some of which I've learned from years of reading the many studies in this field and attending and speaking at hundreds of medical conferences around the world. But more than that, my age-defying principles are based on the experience I've gained from treating more than sixty thousand patients over forty years.

Undoing the Damage

My first age-defying principle is very straightforward. You must undo the damage you've suffered from the dietary mistakes twentieth-century Western civilization has made.

First, you'll need to unlearn the biggest mistake of all—the so-called food pyramid. In the more than ten years since this dietary regime was foisted on the public by our own government, Americans have become fatter than ever. Why? Because the food pyramid is heavily based on carbohydrates of the worst sort: refined grains in the form of bread, pasta, rice, and similar foods. (Not coincidentally in my opinion, these foods are also the ones that are most profitable for the big food processors.) The food pyramid also tells you that protein is bad and fat is worse.

Ignore the food pyramid. Improve your health and prolong your life by cutting carbohydrates from your diet to the degree that is appropriate for you.

Carbohydrate Comprehension

To find the right level of carbohydrates for you, you'll need to understand your own metabolism. If you are overweight, you need to get below your CCLL—your Critical Carbohydrate Level for Losing. You need to stay at that level until you are at your ideal weight. Then you need to find your CCLM—your Critical Carbohydrate Level for Maintenance. Once you've discovered your maintenance carbohydrate level, you need to stay at it for life. I'm certainly not condemning you to a lifetime of dieting and being hungry—I'm helping you make a lifestyle change that will give you better health, more energy, and a longer life. Following my diet for life condemns you only to always feeling satisfied.

If your weight is normal, concern yourself with the nature of your carbohydrates. Most of the carbohydrates you eat should be both complex and unrefined. What does that mean? Complex carbohydrates are basically starchy foods, including whole grains; vegetables such as butternut squash, potatoes, and sweet potatoes; and legumes such as lentils, peas, and beans.

Unrefined applies to the grains. It means whole grains that haven't been so overprocessed that they have no nutritional value. Foods made with unrefined whole grains are hard to come by. The brown-colored commercial bread that passes for "healthy" whole wheat is definitely not what I mean. If you look at the ingredients labels, you'll see that these foods are still made mostly from refined white flour.

Simple carbohydrates are sugars—glucose, sucrose, fructose, lactose, maltose, and so on. Sugars are found in a lot of common foods: milk (lactose), fruit (fructose), beer (maltose), table sugar, sweets, and baked goods such as cake and cookies (sucrose), and soft drinks (corn syrup). These foods have a very high glycemic index (a measure of how quickly and how profoundly the sugars enter your bloodstream) that can send your insulin level soaring. It is essential that you keep simple carbohydrates to the barest possible minimum in your diet. They should be no more than 15 percent of your daily carbohydrate intake. If your daily carbs are no more than 20 percent of your daily diet, that means that simple carbohydrates should be no more than about 3 percent of your daily total. If you must eat something sweet, make it a low-sugar fresh fruit whenever possible. (I'll explain more about how to avoid simple carbohydrates and give you a list of the best fruits to eat in Chapter 21.)

Keep refined carbs (flours, sugars, corn syrup) to less than one serving daily. That means cutting back sharply on pasta, bread, rice, and baked goods, to say nothing of candy and soda pop. I'd be the first to admit that's a big change in diet for most people. But I can also tell you that the very foods that you think you can't live without are usually the ones that will shorten your life. The millions of people who follow my diet plan have gladly given up these foods in exchange for finding improved health and losing weight. Do you love jelly doughnuts so much that you're willing to trade ten years of your life for them? I doubt it.

Carbohydrates for Unstable Blood Sugar

When you digest your food, both simple and complex carbohydrates are converted to glucose, your body's primary energy fuel. The difference is how fast it happens. Complex carbs, especially if they're also high in dietary fiber, take a while to be digested and converted. When you eat these foods, the glucose gets released into your blood slowly and steadily. As your blood sugar slowly rises, your pancreas slowly releases insulin to carry the glucose into your cells. That's why we say these foods have a low glycemic index—the glucose enters your bloodstream slowly.

Sugars, however, are much simpler to digest. They have a very high glycemic index—they enter your bloodstream almost as soon as you swallow them. To cope with the sudden onslaught, your pancreas has to release a lot of insulin all at once. All that insulin mops up all that extra blood glucose so efficiently that your glucose level falls sharply.

If your body can handle glucose normally, and if you eat a mixed meal that includes a variety of foods, the effects on your blood sugar of eating some simple carbohydrates will be relatively benign. Your body will cope with the unneeded sugar efficiently and your blood sugar and insulin levels will return to their normal levels smoothly—for now. As you get older and continue to eat this way, however, your body may become less and less efficient at dealing with the extra glucose.

Unfortunately, nearly half of American adults over age

forty can't handle glucose normally. If you're one of those people—and chances are good you are, especially if you're overweight—your blood glucose levels have roller-coaster ups and
downs. You get all the symptoms of unstable blood sugar, including variable energy levels, mood swings, and cognitive
problems such as fuzzy thinking or brain fog. If the symptoms
come on when you are hungry and are relieved by eating, then
you have the cardinal symptoms of unstable blood sugar.

Do not, by the way, let your conventional doctor do a simple blood test for high blood sugar and tell you that you're fine.
The only way to learn if you have unstable blood sugar is to
have a full, five-hour glucose tolerance test (GTT) administered
by a doctor who knows what he or she is doing.

The Diet to Correct Unstable Blood Sugar

Unstable blood sugar is strictly a diet-related disorder. To control it, never lose sight of these facts:

- *Your blood sugar is destabilized by carbohydrates.*
- *Your blood sugar is basically unaffected by protein.*
- *Your blood sugar is stabilized by dietary fats and oils.*

If unstable blood sugar is a problem for you, a diet low in
carbohydrates and reasonably high in fat is essential to normalize it. This, plus the fact that scientific researchers keep
demonstrating that dietary fats actually contribute to good
health, allows me to recommend a diet having 50 percent of its
calories as fat to my patients with unstable blood sugar. When
they eat a high-fat diet and sharply reduce their carbohydrate
intake, they invariably get better.

Fat Facts

A major part of your antiaging diet must be avoiding the unhealthful fats that have been brought into widespread use in the last century. I'm not talking about the saturated fats such as butter and animal fat that your conventional doctor considers unhealthful. I mean the deadly trans fats that are now found in all sorts of foods, including the margarine your conventional doctor recommends instead of butter.

Trans fats, not saturated fats, are the dietary link to elevated cholesterol and heart disease. Trans fats lower HDL cholesterol, raise LDL cholesterol, raise lipoprotein(a), and raise total cholesterol by 20 to 30 percent. In addition, trans fats reduce your responsiveness to insulin and block your uptake of the essential fatty acids you need for good health.

Select Safe Foods

Most of the prepared and processed foods we eat today are designed more for long shelf life than good nutrition. Most of the nutrients originally present in the fresh version of these foods have been eliminated and replaced with preservatives, food colorings, and all sorts of additives. Avoid these foods. Select unprocessed foods whenever possible. And watch out for "low-fat" foods—the fats in these foods have been replaced by carbohydrates.

Make sure that the majority of animal foods you eat do not contain hormones or antibiotics. Choose hormone-free, antibiotic-free organic meats and free-range poultry and eggs whenever possible. (I realize that, especially in restaurants, these options are not always available.) Today hormone-treated beef is a major international trade issue. European countries have quite rightly banned the import of this meat from America. Rather than rethink the whole issue and realize how unhealthful beef treated in this way is, American trade officials have been fighting the ban in every way they can. It's the food establishment at work again, this time with the overt support of your government, to keep you from getting safer food unless you're willing to pay a premium price for organic meat.

Getting the Most from Your Meals

Make the most of your meals by choosing nutrient-dense foods: foods that have been minimally processed, are high in vitamins, minerals, and phytochemicals, and are low in pesticides, hormones, and antibiotics. Choose the freshest foods you can find, preferably from local suppliers and organic growers. The improvement in the nutrient density with local produce is sometimes remarkable. Whenever I go to Greece, for example, I'm always amazed at the eggs. When they're cooked sunny-side up, the yolks are a magnificent deep yellow-orange color. They taste delicious and have ten times the amount of the vital brain nutrient docosahexaenoic acid (DHA) as do eggs produced on an American factory farm. If you buy organic, free-range eggs from a local farmer, you'll be getting much more nutrition and better taste.

Variety Is the Spice of Health

Despite all my criticisms of the American food industry, it provides us with one advantage that no culture in history has ever had. We now may select from an incredibly wide variety of fresh foods available all year round. Today we can easily

achieve a never-before-imagined selection of different healthful foods in our diets. There are two reasons why this can help
us. First, each food provides us with a different lineup of vitanutrients, thus enhancing the breadth of all food-based nutrition. We know that the phytochemicals in plant foods are very
valuable, but we haven't identified them all yet. By eating a
variety of foods, you get the benefits of the full range of phytochemicals. Second, eating the same food repeatedly has been
shown to create a high incidence of intolerance, or even addic-
tion, to that very food. Now we have the option of choosing
different foods every day.

Fend off Food Allergies

Hidden food intolerances or food allergies are one of the most
common health problems we deal with at the Atkins Center.
It's important that you discover any food intolerances or allergies you have and eliminate those foods from your diet.

Food intolerances often develop simply from eating the
same food too often. Sometimes the food intolerance becomes
fixed enough that several months without that food is necessary. In the case of true allergies, the restriction might be per-
manent.

You can begin to discover your own food intolerance simply by being alert to your reactions to various foods. A common
example is the drowsiness many of my patients feel an hour or
two after eating wheat- or gluten-containing grain foods such
as bread or pasta.

To learn more about any food intolerances or allergies you
have, you'll need to work with a physician, generally one who
practices complementary medicine. The best way to diagnose
intolerances is with a blood specimen using the cytotoxic test

or the **ALCAT**. You'll need to modify your diet based on the results.

Assessing Your Past Diet

The final step is to analyze your dietary history with this book in mind. If you have spent much of your life eating a lot of junk food or avoiding foods that seem now to be contributors to good health, now's the time to start making up the difference. Try to compensate by developing the habit of eating differently enough to correct your previous diet's excesses or inadequacies. That's what I'll be talking about in the next few chapters.

20

The Basic Age-Defying Program

At the Atkins Center we have long worked with two basic sets of dietary instructions. The instructions are very flexible so that we can individualize them for each patient, but basically, one diet induces weight loss regardless of the quantities taken in; the other does not.

Since many of you are already familiar with my basic weight-loss diet, as explained in great detail in *Dr. Atkins' New Diet Revolution*, in this chapter I'll describe my *other* diet, the one that is suitable for people without overt blood sugar or weight problems. This diet applies to only a minority of Americans—over half of all Americans are overweight. If the message of this book is heeded, however, in the future it will apply to most of us, especially those who are fortunate enough to be started on the principles of it from an early age. Why? Because the diet prevents blood sugar problems, high blood pressure, and obesity. More significantly, the diet is based on the foods Americans ate more than a century ago, before heart attacks were ever heard of.

But why, you may be asking, should you go on a diet if you

don't need to lose weight? Because, like practically all other Americans, even those of normal weight, you are at grave risk of developing blood sugar problems later on, if you're not on the brink of such problems already. The reason is the typical junkocentric American diet, which is far too high in refined carbohydrates and far too low in healthful fats, oils, and protein. If you've been faithfully following the government-approved food pyramid for "healthy" eating, you are more than likely to develop unstable blood sugar. This diet calls for you to eat six to eleven servings a day of refined grains such as bread, pasta, and cereals—the junk-food equivalent of swallowing two cups of pure table sugar. That's on top of the 150 pounds of sugar or corn syrup per year (nearly seven ounces a day) that have been measured to be part of the average American's diet.

As you know from reading the earlier chapters of this book, nothing will age your body and mind faster than excess glucose in your blood. By following the healthful, natural, insulin-regulating diet that I'm teaching you, you will, over the long run, keep your blood sugar and insulin levels under control and forestall or even prevent premature aging and serious health problems.

Your Goal: Stable Blood Sugar

My age-defying diet is a successful integration of two major principles. First, employ a diet that corrects the metabolic vulnerabilities that apply uniquely to each individual. Second, the diet must be amply endowed with the vitanutrients most useful in fighting off aging changes.

The first objective is best met by stabilizing the blood sugar to give you the health benefits that flow from keeping the sugar in an optimal range. This is achieved by eliminating most simple carbohydrates and sugar-containing foods and replacing them either with complex carbohydrates or noncarbohydrate food, which leads to the quantities of protein and fats being higher than you may be accustomed to. They are there to stabilize your blood sugar and provide the nutritionally essential amino acids and fatty acids that are as indispensable as vitamins and minerals.

The secondary objective of my age-defying diet is best met by a diet that is low in foods that create free radicals and high in the antioxidants that fight them. To reduce your intake of radical-producing foods, the diet eliminates sugar and trans fats such as margarine from your diet. To increase your antioxidant capacity, the diet is very high in fresh vegetables and low-sugar fruits such as berries.

The great beauty of the age-defying diet is that it is very easy to stick to—it's delicious and you never have to count calories or keep track of your portions. You'll enjoy all the steaks and lobster you want, along with practically unlimited quantities of fresh vegetables. True, sugary foods such as cake and cookies are now permanently out the window, but in their place are a variety of fresh fruits as well as desserts made with natural noncaloric substances much sweeter than sugar. My patients invariably tell me that they lose their taste for sugary foods once they've been on the diet for a couple of weeks. They soon find that typical snacks and desserts are almost disgustingly sweet.

On the age-defying diet your consumption of refined complex carbohydrates such as white rice, bread, and pasta is very limited. In their place are highly nutritious and very flavorful whole grains such as brown rice and genuine whole-grain bread. As with sugary foods, once you start eating whole grains you will soon lose your taste for pasty, flavorless foods made with refined grains.

Components of the Age-Defying Diet

The age-defying diet has three components: protein and fats, complex carbohydrates, and simple carbohydrates. Let's sort the most common foods into their categories and the proportions these foods should contribute to your overall diet:

Proteins and fats: Meat, poultry, eggs, fish, seafood, cheese, nuts, seeds, olives, avocados, fats and oils. The range is 50 to 75 percent.

Complex carbohydrates: Vegetables, grains, whole-grain flour products (pasta, for instance), and legumes (beans). The range is 25 to 50 percent (the lower end is more desirable).

Simple carbohydrates: Fruit, fruit juice, sweets (sugar, honey, maple syrup, etc.), milk, yogurt. The range is less than 10 percent. Whole fruits that are low in sugar content (berries, melons, peaches, plums, apricots, kiwis, and so on) should make up the majority of this category.

Proteins and Fats

To achieve the desirable protein and fat percentages on the age-defying diet, animal foods such as meat, poultry, fish, and shellfish are all permitted in unlimited quantities. Canned fish such as sardines, salmon, and tuna are fine, but be careful of processed meats such as frankfurters and cold cuts. Many of these foods contain hidden carbohydrates such as milk solids or corn syrup as fillers and flavoring. They're also full of undesirable chemical additives such as MSG and nitrates. Just as bad are meats filled with added hormones and antibiotics. To avoid these dangerous additives, whenever possible select "organic" meats. Many meats imported from Argentina or New Zealand are thus qualified.

Eggs are permitted without restriction. Eat the whole egg, not just the whites. As I've pointed out over and over again in this book, eggs are the perfect protein food and contain numerous nutrients that are valuable to your health.

Cheeses are permitted without restriction, because the processing sharply reduces the amount of lactose (milk sugar) in these dairy products. (The exception applies to people who must be on a diet to control yeast overgrowth.) Be sure you're eating real cheese, not a processed cheese food such as Velveeta or American cheese that contains corn oil instead of butterfat.

Milk and yogurt are high in lactose, a simple sugar, and should be kept to a minimum on the age-defying diet. That aside, a significant part of the population can't digest lactose properly or is allergic to milk. Consume no more than one cup of milk daily. Lactose-reduced milk, by the way, has almost exactly the same carbohydrate content as whole milk. If you enjoy yogurt and can digest it easily, eat no more than one cup daily—and eat only the plain, live-culture variety. An eight-ounce container of low-fat, fruit-flavored yogurt contains seven teaspoons of added sugar.

Cream is allowed—in fact, I encourage you to use it. Cream contains very little lactose, but it is an excellent source of dietary fat. Never use nondairy "creamers" or "lighteners." These artificial substances are nothing but sweetened chemicals.

All nuts and seeds are permitted. I personally recommend macadamia nuts. These tasty, crunchy nuts are high in healthy monosaturated fat and low in carbohydrate. They're the perfect snack food. Other good nut choices are pecans, filberts, and walnuts. Nut butters are permitted—but only if they contain no added sweeteners or partially hydrogenated vegetable oils. That leaves out many commercial peanut butters. Check your local health food store for nut butters with no additives.

Fats and oils are nutritionally essential, no matter what the

American Heart Association and the rest of the medical establishment tell you. They should never be avoided or feared—with one exception. That's the dangerous trans fats. If the label on the food container says "partially hydrogenated vegetable oil," stay away. Your conventional doctor may well have told you to stop eating butter and switch to more healthful margarine. Don't you believe it! Exactly the opposite is true. Although the newer margarines are somewhat less constructed of trans fats, they still represent the greatest source of these most unhealthful fats. Eating this stuff promises to release cascades of artery-damaging free radicals as your body tries to cope with it. Butter doesn't do this. It not only gives your food a richer, more satisfying taste, it is a rather safe form of fat. All fats, butter included, help stabilize your blood sugar.

For salads and cooking, monounsaturated vegetable oils such as olive, almond, avocado, and macadamia are ideal. Cold-pressed polyunsaturated vegetable oils, such as walnut, soy, sesame, sunflower, and safflower, are also fine. These oils are excellent dietary sources of omega-3 and omega-6 essential fatty acids. Skip the corn oil and the canola oil—they're far too high in omega-6.

Complex Carbohydrates

Now we're at the part of the age-defying diet that distinguishes it from the Atkins weight-loss diet. Here we allow carbohydrates, but they must be those that contribute most to your health. The first technique is to replace the simple carbohydrates (sugars) in your diet with high-quality complex carbohydrates (starches). Simple sugars send your blood sugar crashing up and down. Complex carbohydrates are more likely to keep your blood sugar steady, especially when you combine them with protein and fat.

Notice my emphasis on the word "high-quality" when discussing complex carbohydrates. Foods such as white rice, pasta, and bread are, technically speaking, complex carbohydrates, but their quality is very low. The grains used to make these foods have been processed to the point of nutritional nonexistence. The phytonutrients and fiber in them have been removed, leaving behind nothing but refined, concentrated carbohydrates—carbohydrates your body converts almost instantly to glucose.

The age-defying diet emphasizes the high-quality complex carbohydrates found in whole grains, nuts, seeds, and vegetables. These foods are delicious, filling, and full of fiber, vitamins, minerals, and phytonutrients that fight free radicals and have other beneficial effects.

On the age-defying diet, if it's green, it's a relatively free food (unless a weight problem or blood sugar disorder causes you to be better off on a relatively low-carbohydrate diet). This means generous and varied portions of salad greens, broccoli, kale, brussels sprouts, collard greens, green beans, and so on. This may come to four to six cups a day.

Other vegetables such as carrots, beets, peas, and winter squash are higher in carbohydrates, but they're also high in antioxidant carotenes and other nutrients. To get the benefits of the phytochemicals without overdoing the carbohydrates, refer to the tables in Chapter 21 and select those vegetables that provide significant amounts of phytochemicals without a major intake of carbohydrates.

Starchy vegetables, beans and legumes, corn, and even potatoes can be useful sources of vegetable protein, essential fatty acids, fiber, vitanutrients, and phytochemicals. On the other hand, because they are relatively high in starch (which your body converts to glucose), they could raise your blood sugar, especially if you tend even slightly in that direction. Because these foods are also high in fiber, however, the rise in blood sugar they cause is slower and far less dramatic than eating an equivalent amount of refined carbohydrates such as pasta.

I find that my patients need to experiment a bit to find the level of complex carbohydrates that is right for them. In general, if you are normal weight, you should limit starchy vegetables such as potatoes, beans, and similar foods, to one or two servings a day. However, if you find yourself losing weight on the age-defying diet, add another serving or two. People who are underweight should fill up on vegetables. This may include three to four servings of these complex carbohydrates a day.

As you permanently change your eating habits, you'll discover the amount of complex carbohydrates that satisfies you and also keeps your weight and blood sugar at the appropriate level. You can even allow yourself the occasional little binge, as long as you stick to bingeing on high-quality carbohydrates. If you want to have a small serving of pasta, for instance, you may—as long as you make it whole-wheat pasta or buckwheat noodles. If you'd like some rice, brown rice is certainly better than white. A small baked potato with the skin and some sour cream is actually better than a dry baked potato—and certainly better than a serving of french fries.

Simple Carbohydrates

If you're overweight, I have a very simple method for determining how many simple carbohydrates to include in your diet. Just follow these easy steps: Take a piece of paper. Take a pencil. Draw a large circle on the paper. Read the answer. That's a zero.

If you're normal weight, you still want to keep simple carbohydrates and highly refined complex carbohydrates such as pasta, bread, and sugary foods to a bare minimum. Not only are these foods very high on the glycemic index, they've been heavily processed and have very little nutritional value—they are the emptiest of empty calories.

What about fresh fruit? There is a place for it, but it is not the unrestricted benefactor many dietitians today believe it to be. Bear in mind that most of the calories in fruit come from the simple sugars fructose and glucose—the very sugars present in white table sugar. The other side of the coin is that fruit is a useful source of fiber, vitamins, minerals, and phytonutrients. If you're of normal weight, fresh whole fruits in modest amounts can be acceptable. You must learn which fruits provide the greatest phytochemical and vitanutrient intake in relation to their sugar content. Table 21.2 in Chapter 21 should help you make good selections. You will see that the greatest advantage comes from berries of all sorts, backed up by melons, peaches, plums, apricots, and kiwi.

Fruit juices are most assuredly *not* a good alternative to fruit and should be avoided. The juicing process removes the fiber and concentrates the sugar. For example, orange juice, for all that it is heavily advertised as an excellent source of vitamin C, folic acid, potassium, and other vitanutrients, is also extremely high in sugar. One 8-ounce serving has more than 25 grams of sugar in it—more than the average candy bar. Apple juice, grape juice, pineapple juice, and prune juice all have even more. Among the vegetable juices, carrot juice is very high in sugar and should be avoided by itself. It would be appropriate only as a minor addition to mixed vegetable juices. On the other hand, tomato juice is definitely worth your effort. A 6-ounce glass of tomato juice (even the processed kind out of the bottle) contains enough lycopene to make a difference.

Canned fruits have virtually no nutritional value, and they are loaded with added sugar. The same is true of dried fruit, such as raisins, prunes, and dried pineapple. Sugar or some other sweetener is often added in the processing, even if the product is advertised as "healthy," "organic," or "natural."

As for other simple sugars, the short answer is no. The long answer is—if you're addicted to sweets—no. If you're not, then you can have simple sugars once in a leap year blue moon. You need to avoid all caloric sweeteners, including table sugar, honey, maple syrup, corn syrup, fructose, maltose (found in beer, even the nonalcoholic kind), and lactose (milk sugar). Basically, if the food ends in *-ose*, it's a sugar and should be avoided.

If you feel the need for something sweet, select or create a rich dessert sweetened by a noncaloric sweetener. The two most desirable alternative sweeteners available today are stevia and sucralose. Stevia is a natural plant product from South America that has been used safely worldwide for years. The stevia herb in its natural form is about ten to fifteen times sweeter than table sugar. Stevia extracts are much sweeter, some one hundred to three hundred times sweeter than table sugar, so a tiny bit goes a long way. Sucralose has just been approved by the FDA for use in the United States. It is derived from table sugar, but sucralose is six hundred times sweeter, plus it is absorbed into your body only in limited amounts. That means your overworked insulin mechanism need not be involved.

A few years ago the FDA, in one of its many misguided attempts to "protect" American consumers, succeeded in making the publisher of a cookbook of stevia recipes destroy them. Public outrage could not stop the strong-arm tactics, and to this day stevia can be sold only in health food stores as a food additive. It can't be labeled as the natural sweetener it is.

Stevia or sucralose is a much better choice for a noncaloric sweetener than aspartame (Nutra-Sweet™ or Equal™), an artificial sweetener that often seems to cause side effects, especially headaches, in many of my patients. In addition, my patients who were taking in large quantities (three or more servings a day) of aspartame-sweetened foods or beverages seemed to have trouble losing weight and controlling their blood sugar. They achieved success only after they changed to other noncaloric sweeteners.

Drink Up

Drinking enough fluids is an important aspect of the age-defying diet. Consume liquids liberally, but don't force yourself. Your goal should be to drink at least eight 8-ounce glasses (two quarts) of fluid a day. Plain, pure water is the most natural and best of all liquids to drink. If at all possible, it should be bottled spring or mineral water or tap water from an effective water filtration system. Plain sodium-free seltzer and essence-flavored unsweetened seltzers are also fine. You can make your own lemonade with fresh lemon juice, pure water, and a noncaloric sweetener such as stevia.

Herbal teas, when made with pure water, are an enjoyable alternative to plain water. Choose herbal teas that are free of caffeine, added sweeteners, fruit, and barley malt. Good choices are peppermint, chamomile, and raspberry leaf.

Decaffeinated coffee and tea are allowed (the water-based decaffeination process is recommended). Caffeine stimulates insulin production, causing your blood sugar to first rise and then crash. If you're vulnerable to unstable blood sugar, this

could result in fatigue, irritability, and cravings for carbohydrates. Try eliminating caffeine from your diet for a couple of
weeks and see how you feel. If you notice that your energy levels even out, caffeine definitely affects your blood sugar and
should be avoided.

As I explained earlier, green tea is an excellent source of
antioxidant flavonoids. I recommend at least two cups a day.
Green tea is considerably lower in caffeine than coffee or even
black tea. Decaffeinated green tea is now available, but so few
people are troubled by the caffeine in green tea that it is rarely
necessary.

What about alcoholic beverages? Several studies have
shown that having a drink a day, especially a glass of red wine,
has a beneficial effect on the heart. If you're already in the habit
of having a daily cocktail or glass of wine with dinner, if your
weight is normal, and if you have no blood sugar instability,
then you are well off to continue to have your daily drink.
Those are a lot of ifs, and I find that nearly half of my patients
should not be drinking alcohol at all. When you drink alcohol,
stick to dry wine or straight liquor with a sugarless mixer such
as seltzer or diet soda. Avoid beer and dessert wines.

How Much Should I Eat?

While you've been reading this chapter you might have been
wondering what I mean by a serving. After all, other diet books
tell you exactly how much of each food to eat, down to the last
ounce. Those of you who have read my earlier books already
know that I take the opposite approach. Counting calories and
portions has very little to do with a diet that will help you live
to a ripe old age. That is, as long as you remain at your ideal
weight.

My general rule is to eat the amount that makes you feel comfortable. That's the amount—whatever it may be—that satisfies your hunger with a variety of delicious foods. You'll find that by cutting out the simple carbohydrates from your diet, and substituting protein, fats, and complex carbohydrates, your appetite is quickly satisfied without even having to think about calories, much less count them. Overeating becomes almost impossible.

How often you eat is just as important as what you eat. Try to start each day with a large, high-protein breakfast—a cheese omelette, for example. Eating at least three full meals a day is essential for keeping your blood sugar steady. Many of my patients find they actually do better on four to six smaller meals a day, including a protein snack before bed. Remember, the quality of your food counts more than the quantity.

You've now learned the principles of my age-defying diet, but it will take a little more explaining to tell you how to personalize it so that it matches *your* metabolism, *your* health vulnerabilities, and *your* food preferences.

By the time you finish the next chapter, I expect that you will know pretty much exactly how you can do it.

21

Living the Age-Defying Way

Let's start this chapter with a pop quiz. How much sugar does the average American eat each day? I think you'll be amazed by the answer: twenty teaspoons. That's twenty of those little sugar packets, or nearly four ounces, or almost half a cup. Sugar consumption has increased 28 percent since 1983. In the form of table sugar, high-fructose corn syrup, or other caloric sweeteners, sugar now accounts for 16 percent of the calories consumed by the average American. Even worse, sugar is now 20 percent of teenagers' calories.[1]

Here's another quiz question: How many adult Americans are overweight? Some ninety-seven million people, or 55 percent of the population.[2]

Could there possibly be any connection? Not if you ask the U.S. Department of Agriculture, the wonderful people who brought you the infamous food pyramid. According to them, ten teaspoons of sugar a day are just fine. I wonder if that much sugar is what they mean when they tell you in the food pyramid to use sugar sparingly.

In this chapter I'm going to teach you how to throw the

food pyramid out the window and select the foods you should eat for a long and healthy life. The very first food you're going to throw out the window is sugar, followed immediately by the refined carbohydrates that are the basis of the food pyramid. As I've discussed throughout this book, nothing will age you faster than a diet high in carbohydrates.

Your Ideal Carbohydrate Level

In the previous chapters you learned how important it is to keep your carbohydrate consumption low. How low? Remember my cardinal rule: One diet does not fit all. You now need to discover the most liberal level of carbohydrate consumption that corresponds to your own individual metabolism and keeps you at your normal weight.

In this chapter, I will start with the less-than-probable assumption that you are of normal weight or even underweight or have achieved normal weight through successful dieting. This allows me to teach you how to differentiate those carbohydrates most likely to make you healthier from those which have been creating epidemics of diabetes, heart disease, and shortened life spans.

Those of you with a weight problem, even if it is under control through dieting, will need this information even more, because in order both to achieve your ideal weight and stay there, you will have to find the nutritional elements of healthful carbohydrates from a relatively low number of total carbohydrates.

The most essential element in dealing with your carbohydrate intake is obtaining an accurate estimate of what your total daily allowance of carbohydrates should be. In *Dr. Atkins' New Diet Revolution,* which I urge you to read and follow if you are overweight, I taught that there are two levels of daily carbohydrate intake that must be identified for each individual. One applies only to overweight people; I gave it the name Critical Carbohydrate Level for Losing (CCLL). This is the number of daily grams of carbohydrate intake below which there is automatic weight loss. The other level applies to everyone. I gave it the name Critical Carbohydrate Level for Maintenance (CCLM). This is the carbohydrate intake level above which you will gain weight.

For those few of you who simply do not gain weight, I must change the term to read Ideal Carbohydrate Level for Maintenance (ICLM), because your goal is health preservation, not weight control.

If you have a weight-gaining tendency, your personal CCLM could be anywhere from 25 to 90 grams of carbohydrates a day. How can you know what your daily carbohydrate intake should be within that fairly broad range? Well, every person is different, but if you've already lost weight on my low-carbohydrate diet, you have a good idea of what the right level is for you, based on what you had to do to lose weight. In general, restrict your carbohydrates to 60 grams to start and see how you do. If you have real difficulty losing weight and need to sharply restrict your carbohydrate intake, your CCLM will be even lower, probably between 25 and 40 grams a day. People who lose weight relatively easily will probably end up with a carbohydrate intake between 40 and 60 grams a day. People who lose weight easily will probably find that between 60 and 90 carbohydrate grams a day is good for them.

But even if you've never had a weight problem, you're not off the carbohydrate hook. To defy the aging process, you must still keep your carbohydrates to the lowest amount consistent with feeling your best. For you, that may add up to 90 to 150 grams a day. Remember, your goal here is not weight loss, it's the prevention of health problems related to aging. A major part of those problems is related to excess carbohydrate consumption, even among people of normal weight.

These carbohydrate gram counts are simply guidelines, however. If your weight starts to creep up on 60 grams of carbohydrates a day, then clearly you must cut back to the level that keeps your weight steady. Conversely, if you start to lose weight on 60 grams a day, it's an opportunity to add one or two servings of health-providing carbohydrates each day.

The main reason I suggest keeping carbohydrate intake low, even without a weight problem, is the fact that keeping your blood sugar stable is also very important to defying aging. To do this, the restriction of carbohydrates, especially refined ones, is important.

Balancing Carbohydrates

The age-defying diet has two main pillars: Eat foods low in carbohydrates and high in antioxidants. It is crucial to balance the two. Fortunately, many of the best low-carbohydrate foods are also very high in artery-protecting, cancer-fighting antioxidants such as carotenoids.

How high? In recent years some extremely interesting research has been done that tells us exactly which vegetables and fruits are the best to eat. In these studies, individual foods have been carefully analyzed using a sophisticated assay technique that can accurately measure their total antioxidant capacity.[3]

The pioneering effort began at the Jean Mayer USDA Human Nutrition Center on Aging at Tufts University, and I find this sort of work very heartening. Perhaps our own government will eventually come to realize the folly of the food pyramid and recognize that significant work done by its own scientists points in another, much more healthful direction.

At the Atkins Center, we have taken this extremely important research a step further. By looking at both the antioxidant scores of common vegetables and fruits and their carbohydrate content, we have been able to determine the ratio of antioxidant value to carbohydrate grams, a figure I call the Atkins Ratio. The higher the Atkins Ratio, the more antioxidant protection you get per gram of carbohydrate. As a general rule, foods with an Atkins Ratio of 2 or more are the most desirable. With the Atkins Ratios, you now have a scientifically accurate way to choose the foods that are best for you.

Let's start with vegetables. Table 21.1 ranks popular vegetables in descending order of antioxidant protection and gives their antioxidant score. (The score is based on a complex formula that compares the antioxidant capacity of the vegetable to a standard called the Trolox equivalent.) The chart also lists the carbohydrate content of a typical serving of the vegetable and gives you the Atkins Ratio.

As you can see, you get the most antioxidant protection per typical serving from garlic and kale, and the least protection from celery and cucumbers. When you look at the Atkins Ratio, however, you easily see that some foods that are high on the antioxidant scale are also high in carbohydrates and therefore have a low ratio. Corn, for instance, is 7.2 on the antioxidant scale, but there are 20.6 grams of carbohydrate in a half-cup serving. That makes the ratio of antioxidant protection to carbohydrates a low 0.3. Overall, the starchier a vegetable is, the lower its ratio of antioxidant protection to carbohydrates. Sweet potatoes, for instance, are often touted as being particularly healthful because of their high beta-carotene content. In fact, as the table shows, sweet potatoes aren't particularly high in antioxidants relative to other vegetables. They are very high

TABLE 21.1

Total Antioxidant Capacity of Common Vegetables

Vegetable	Antioxidant Score (per serving)*	Carbohydrates (in grams)	Atkins Ratio
Kale	24.1	3.7	6.5
Garlic (1 clove)	23.2	1.0	23.2
Spinach	17.0	3.4	5.0
Brussels sprouts	15.8	6.8	2.3
Broccoli	12.9	4.0	3.2
Beets	11.7	5.7	2.1
Red bell pepper (raw)	8.1	3.2	2.5
Corn	7.2	20.6	0.3
Onion (1 tablespoon)	5.6	0.9	6.2
Eggplant	5.1	3.2	1.6
Cauliflower	5.1	2.9	1.8
Cabbage	4.8	4.0	1.2
Potato (1 whole)	4.6	51.0	0.09
Sweet potato	4.3	27.7	0.15
Leaf lettuce (1 leaf)	4.1	0.5	8.2
Green beans	3.9	4.9	0.8
Carrots	3.4	8.2	0.4
Yellow squash	2.8	3.9	0.7
Iceberg lettuce (1 leaf)	2.3	0.4	5.8
Celery (raw)	1.1	0.75	1.5
Cucumber (raw)	1.1	1.5	0.7

*Serving is one-half cup cooked unless otherwise indicated.

SOURCES: Cao, G., E. Sofic, and R. L. Prior. "Antioxidant Capacity of Tea and Common Vegetables." *Journal of Agricultural and Food Chemistry* 44 (1996): 3426–31; Pennington, Jean A. T., ed. *Bowes & Church's Food Values of Portions Commonly Used.* 16th ed. Philadelphia: Lippincott, 1994.

in carbohydrates, however—a typical baked sweet potato contains nearly 28 grams. The Atkins Ratio for a sweet potato is only 0.15. If you're only going to eat 40 grams of carbohydrates a day, then, you'd be much better off eating foods that give you a higher Atkins Ratio, such as greens, broccoli, red bell peppers, and so on.

The vegetables listed in the tables are those for which we have scientifically established antioxidant values—research in this area is still in the early stages and not all vegetables have been analyzed yet. Vegetables not on the list are not precluded—just avoid the starchy ones whenever you can. By eating a variety of vegetables, you avoid being bored by your food. You also avoid the possibility of developing food sensitivities from eating the same few foods day in and day out.

Take Time for Tea

The antioxidant capacity of an eight-ounce cup of freshly brewed green tea is anywhere from four to five times as great as a serving of kale. For black tea (the kind found in most tea bags), the antioxidant capacity is almost as high. As I discussed earlier, the phenols in tea are powerful antioxidants that have been shown to help prevent cancer, among other benefits. I strongly recommend at least one cup of freshly brewed tea a day as part of your antiaging diet. Make the tea using pure water and sweeten it, if you wish, only with noncaloric sweeteners such as saccharin, stevia, or sucralose. Most important, do not add milk or cream to your tea. The proteins in the milk will bind with the phenols in the tea and keep you from absorbing them.

Favorite Fruits

The same analytical techniques applied to vegetables have been applied to a variety of fruits. The results tell us exactly which fruits have the highest Atkins Ratio, as listed in Table 21.2.

As with the vegetables, the fruits that are highest in antioxi-

TABLE 21.2

Total Antioxidant Capacity of Common Fruits

Fruit	Antioxidant Score (per serving)*	Carbohydrates (in grams)	Atkins Ratio
Blueberries	24.0	10.3	2.3
Blackberries	20.0	9.2	2.2
Strawberries	12.4	5.3	2.3
Plum	8.4	8.6	1.0
Orange	6.8	8.2	0.8
Kiwi	5.5	11.3	0.5
Pink grapefruit	4.5	9.5	0.5
Red grapes	3.9	7.9	0.5
Green grapes	2.9	7.9	0.4
Banana	2.1	13.4	0.2
Apple	1.9	10.5	0.2
Tomato	1.6	2.9	0.5
Pear	1.2	12.5	0.1
Honeydew melon	0.9	7.8	0.1

*Serving is one-half cup raw.

sources: Wang, H., G. Cao, and R. L. Prior. "Total Antioxidant Capacity of Fruits." *Journal of Agricultural and Food Chemistry* 44 (1996): 701–05; Prior, R. L. et al. "Antioxidant Capacity as Influenced by Total Phenolic and Anthocyanin Content, Maturity, and Variety of *Vaccinium* Species." *Journal of Agricultural and Food Chemistry* 46 (1998): 2686–93; Pennington, Jean A. T., ed. *Bowes & Church's Food Values of Portions Commonly Used.* 16th ed. Philadelphia: Lippincott, 1994.

dant protection turn out to be the ones that are also lowest in carbohydrates. Blueberries, the top antioxidant fruit with a ranking of 24, have only 10 grams of carbohydrate in half a cup, and thus an Atkins Ratio of 2.3. Compare that to a banana, which has 13 grams of carbohydrate and an antioxidant ranking of just 2.1 in a half cup. Its Atkins Ratio is 0.2. It's obvious that blueberries are by far the better choice.

You might think that if a fruit is a good source of antioxidants, then fruit juice, which is more concentrated, would be better. That's only partially true. In the case of commercial grape juice, which is made using dark-skinned purple grapes, the antioxidant level is indeed higher, mostly because purple (Concord) grapes have more flavonoids. Tomato juice also has a higher antioxidant score than fresh tomatoes. Orange juice and apple juice, however, have much lower antioxidant scores than the fresh fruit. Overall, select whole fruits and avoid fruit juices.

Relatively speaking, vegetables have considerably more antioxidant value per carbohydrate gram than fruits and thus represent a much more valuable dietary choice. Even so, if your weight is under control, it is not inappropriate for you to use some of your daily carbohydrate ration to eat one or two cups of fruit a day. We have yet to identify all the valuable phytochemicals, or even all the antioxidants in foods, so it makes sense to eat as wide a variety of fresh fruits and vegetables as possible to give yourself the maximum protection.

If you crave something sweet for dessert or a snack, fruit is certainly a better choice than a candy bar or cookies. The lower glycemic index of some fruits means that your blood sugar stays steadier. Even so, sugar is sugar and should be kept to a minimum by selecting lower-carbohydrate fruits whenever possible.

As I indicated, your best choices among the fruits are berries of any kind. A dish of blueberries or strawberries, topped with whipped cream or mixed with ricotta cheese sweetened with stevia or sucralose, is one of my favorite desserts. One word of caution: Frozen berries are almost as high in antioxidants as fresh, but they may have added sugar. Read the label carefully and choose a brand that does not.

Half a cup of blueberries has about 10 grams of carbohydrate. Other good low-sugar fruit choices are apricots, peaches, plums, strawberries, honeydew, and cantaloupe. Don't forget that technically speaking, avocados and tomatoes are fruits. Avocados are an excellent source of monounsaturated fat; try to find California avocados, which are much lower in carbohydrates than those from Florida (12 grams to 27).

Counting Carotenoids

I've already discussed the incredible importance of carotenoids such as beta-carotene and lycopene for your health (check back to Chapter 10 for more information). Here I'm going to get specific about the carotenoid content of common fruits and vegetables. Table 21.3 lists the top nineteen carotenoid foods and gives the ratio of carotenoids to carbohydrates.

The best sources of carotenoids in foods are dark-green leafy vegetables and orange-colored foods such as carrots. As you can see from the table, the high carbohydrate content of carrots is outweighed by their very high carotenoid content—the carotenoid/carbohydrate ratio is 11.3. But collard greens are an even better choice, with a carotenoid/carbohydrate ratio of 32.4. For just about half the carbohydrates of carrots, collard greens give you nearly three times the antioxidant protection. Which will you choose? I think the answer is pretty obvious.

Cooking high-carotenoid foods actually increases their nutritional value by breaking down the tough cell walls and

TABLE 21.3

Carotenoids in Fruits and Vegetables

Food	Carotenoid Content (in mcg per g)	Carbohydrates (in grams)	C/C Ratio
Kale	220.0	3.7	59.5
Turnip greens	130.2	1.6	81.4
Collards	126.2	3.9	32.4
Spinach	122.9	3.4	36.1
Sweet potato	94.8	27.7	3.4
Carrots	92.5	8.2	11.3
Butternut squash	57.0	10.7	5.3
Red bell pepper (raw)	46.4	3.2	14.5
Swiss chard	40.0	3.6	11.1
Romaine lettuce (raw)	39.1	0.7	55.8
Tomato (raw)	36.6	2.9	12.6
Broccoli	32.7	4.0	8.2
Apricots (raw)	25.5	7.9	3.2
Zucchini	25.4	3.5	7.3
Brussels sprouts	20.5	6.8	3.0
Cantaloupe (raw)	16.6	6.7	2.5
Green beans	13.4	4.9	2.7
Endive (raw)	9.6	0.8	12.0
Corn	9.5	20.6	0.5

NOTES: Carotenoid figures are total carotenoid content, including alpha-carotene, beta-carotene, lutein, zeaxanthin, lycopene. Portions are one-half cup cooked unless noted otherwise.

SOURCES: USDA–NCC Carotenoid Database for U.S. Foods. 1998: Pennington, Jean A. T., ed. *Bowes & Church's Food Values of Portions Commonly Used.* 16th ed. Philadelphia: Lippincott, 1994.

releasing the carotenoids, especially the beta-carotene. To preserve the other nutrients, however, cook vegetables gently by steaming them in as little water as possible or by sautéing them lightly in olive oil or butter.

One of the carotenoids, lycopene, has been shown to help prevent cancer, particularly prostate cancer. The best dietary source of lycopene is tomatoes. Processing releases the lycopene in tomatoes, so tomato juice or puree has considerably more lycopene than an uncooked tomato. Lycopene is best absorbed by your body if the tomatoes are eaten with some dietary fat, such as olive oil or cheese. Table 21.4 lists the best sources for lycopene in foods and gives the ratio of lycopene to carbohydrates for each. Stay away from tomato ketchup—it's approximately one-third sugar. As the table shows, tomato foods are high in carbohydrates. You may want to take lycopene supplements instead.

TABLE 21.4

Lycopene Content of Foods

Food	Serving Size	Lycopene	Carbohydrates	L/C
Tomato puree	1 cup	35.6	25.1	1.4
Tomato juice	1 cup	25.0	10.3	2.4
Watermelon	1 medium slice	14.7	11.5	1.3
Tomato paste	2 tablespoons	13.8	6.2	2.2
Tomato soup, condensed	1 cup	9.7	22.4	0.4
Pink grapefruit	one half	4.9	9.5	0.5
Tomato, raw	1 medium	3.7	5.7	0.6
Tomato ketchup	1 tablespoon	2.7	4.1	0.7

SOURCES: USDA–NCC Carotenoid Database for U.S. Foods. 1998: Pennington, Jean A. T., ed. *Bowes & Church's Food Values of Portions Commonly Used.* 16th ed. Philadelphia: Lippincott, 1994.

Lutein and zeaxanthin, carotenoids found in vegetables and eggs, are crucial for protecting your eyesight from age-related macular degeneration. Because the two nutrients are hard to break out in analysis, and because you need them both, Table 21.5 lists the top lutein/zeaxanthin foods and gives the lutein/zeaxanthin-to-carbohydrate ratio.

The Value of Fruits and Vegetables

A bedrock principle of alternative medicine is that diet plays a crucial role in health. As a complementary practitioner, I know from my own experience with thousands of patients and from avidly reading numerous studies from Europe and even the United States that those who consume a diet rich in fresh fruits and vegetables have significantly better health profiles than those who eat other carbohydrates. (No study to date, however, has compared fruit and vegetable consumers to subjects whose total carbohydrate intake is extremely low.)

For example, a 1996 meta-analysis looked at well over two hundred studies on the relationship between vegetable and fruit consumption and the risk of cancer. Their conclusion is impressive: There is strong evidence for a protective effect against cancer from these foods.[4] Their conclusion might also have read: Carbohydrates from sources other than fruits and vegetables make cancer more probable.

An interesting recent study compared cardiac risk factors in men from Czechoslovakia, where the death rate from coronary heart disease is high, to men in Germany, where the coronary death rate is moderate, and Israel, where the coronary death rate is low. Most of the traditional indicators, such as cholesterol, were about the same for all three groups. The Czech men, however, had very low levels of carotenoids

TABLE 21.5

Lutein and Zeaxanthin Content of Foods

Food	Lutein/Zeaxanthin (in mcg per g)	Carbohydrates (in grams)	LZ/C ratio
Kale	158.0	3.7	42.7
Turnip greens	84.4	1.6	52.7
Collard greens	80.9	3.9	20.7
Spinach	70.4	3.4	20.7
Romaine lettuce (raw)	26.3	0.7	37.6
Broccoli	22.3	4.0	5.6
Zucchini	21.2	3.5	6.1
Corn	18.0	20.6	0.9
Peas	13.5	12.5	1.1
Brussels sprouts	12.9	6.8	1.9
Green beans	7.0	4.9	1.4
Okra	3.9	5.8	0.7
Orange (raw)	1.8	8.2	0.2
Tomato (raw)	1.3	2.9	7.1
Peach (raw)	0.6	4.9	0.1

NOTE: Portion is one-half cup cooked unless otherwise noted.

SOURCE: USDA–NCC Carotenoid Database for U.S. Foods. 1998; Pennington, Jean A. T., ed. *Bowes & Church's Food Values of Portions Commonly Used.* 16th ed. Philadelphia: Lippincott, 1994.

compared to the Israeli men. The average Czech man had a beta-carotene level of 60 mcg, while his Israeli counterpart had 102 mcg; for lycopene, the numbers were 84 mcg to 223 mcg. Why the difference? The Czech men ate very few fresh fruits and vegetables.[5]

Other researchers have recently studied precisely how much eating fresh fruits and vegetables increases your antioxidant level. In one study, thirty-six healthy people ate a controlled diet for two weeks that included ten or more portions a day of fresh fruits and vegetables. Blood tests showed that the diet significantly increased the total antioxidant capacity of their blood.[6] Another study of elderly women showed that their antioxidant levels were increased when they consumed strawberries, spinach, red wine, or vitamin C—four hours later, their blood antioxidant levels had jumped by anywhere from 7 to 25 percent from the foods.[7]

The Whole Story

One of the unfounded accusations that's often leveled against the Atkins Diet is that it forbids carbohydrates such as bread, pasta, rice, and beans, to say nothing of fruits and vegetables. During the induction phase of my weight-loss diet, that's true— such carbohydrates are indeed prohibited. Once you reach your maintenance weight, however, and have determined the level of carbohydrate intake that works for you, these foods can come back into your life to a greater or lesser extent. Let me stress again, however, that the more carbohydrates you eat, the faster you will age.

Those of you without gluten intolerance should make the most of the carbohydrates in your diet by eating unrefined whole grains. Bread made with genuine whole wheat (not the

brown-colored stuff that passes for whole wheat in most commercial breads) has more gourmet appeal than the enriched
white-flour variation. It's somewhat lower in carbohydrates
than commercial bread and certainly more satisfying. Because
the whole grains still have their bran (the outer coating on the
grain), the bread has a lower glycemic index and much more
nutrition, including all the crucial B vitamins.

Food Intolerances

At the Atkins Center we often find that food allergies underlie
numerous chronic health problems. Many of our patients turn
out to be sensitive to the gluten in wheat and other grains such
as rye, barley, and oats. I attribute the dramatic improvement
in these patients to the elimination of gluten grains from their
diet. (Although of course we improve their nutrition in a variety of other ways as well.)

The easiest way to find out if gluten is a problem for you is
simply to stay away from foods that contain the aforementioned grains. That's certainly not a hardship if you're following the age-defying diet. If your ICLM allows you to have more
carbohydrates in your diet, substitute beans, brown rice, mil-
let, and other gluten-free grains.

Even though unrefined whole grains are generally a little
lower in carbohydrates than their refined counterparts, the difference is slight. Plus, you won't find many high-quality whole-
grain products in your supermarket. Even well-stocked health
food stores carry a lot of products that claim to be made from
whole grains but really aren't. Read the ingredients labels carefully.

I much prefer to see my patients who are eligible for more
carbohydrates add potatoes, yams, succotash, lentils, and the

like instead of grains to their diet. The human digestive tract is simply not well designed for digesting grains. The proteins in grain, especially the gluten, are very difficult to digest, even if you don't have apparent gluten problems. Too much grain, especially of the highly refined kind, is behind many of the cases of food allergies, irritable bowel, chronic indigestion, and yeast overgrowth that I see every day.

Beans and legumes such as kidney beans, chickpeas, and lentils are fairly high in carbohydrates, but I feel that their high vegetable protein content, high fiber content, and beneficial vitanutrient content place them among the better additions to an age-defying diet.

Adding Vitanutrients

This chapter's conclusion is that when carbohydrates are added, your best choices are a variety of fresh vegetables plus fresh fruits in smaller amounts and that these foods should be chosen with an awareness of their Atkins Ratio. The broad array of antioxidants found in these foods is much more valuable for protecting you from free radical damage than is any one supplemental vitanutrient such as vitamin C. Vitanutrient supplements are nonetheless still an important part of your age-defying diet, as I've explained throughout this book.

22

Your Age-Defying
Vitanutrient Plan

In this chapter I give you some basic guidelines for the vitanutrient supplements that will help you defy age. To my
great pleasure, breakthroughs and new developments happen
practically every day in this field. The mere fact that serious
studies of vitanutrients are now commonplace is very encouraging to me and my many colleagues in the area of complementary medicine. The incontrovertible results of these studies
are making it harder and harder for the medical establishment
to ignore them, especially when statistics show that adverse
drug reactions directly cause over one hundred thousand
deaths a year and are implicated in many more. Throughout
this book I've tried to incorporate the latest findings and to pass
on to you my most recent experiences with the many new vitanutrients that are now available.

I've discussed the importance of various vitanutrients for
maintaining and improving your health. The goal is to help you
achieve your maximum life expectancy with minimum disability. Just as no one diet fits all, however, vitanutrient needs vary
from person to person and also change somewhat throughout

your lifetime. After I give you a basic vitamin and mineral formula that's appropriate for almost all adults, I go on to give suggestions for specific health issues. The purpose of so doing is to give you the basis of a flexible supplement program appropriate for most people.

There's no need to purchase each individual supplement and take each one separately. I have developed a prototypical formula for my Atkins Center patients that is also available at health food stores. Many reputable manufacturers now make well-designed formulas that include many or most of the basic vitanutrients in dosages large enough to be effective. In addition, many reputable manufacturers make formulas for treating specific health issues, such as osteoporosis or high blood pressure, just as I do at the Atkins Center. Select a supplement that gives you the maximum breadth and dosage possible, and add whatever other individual vitanutrients that are appropriate for your own physical and medical profile.

I don't have the space here to provide detailed discussions of each of the vitanutrients listed. Many have been discussed earlier in the book, and for detailed information, please see *Dr. Atkins' Vita-Nutrient Solution*.

Basic Vitanutrients

The formula listed in Table 22.1 is designed as a basic nutrition vitamin/mineral formula for adults. When selecting a combined vitamin/mineral supplement, bear in mind that outdated and pointless FDA regulations limit the amount of folic acid to 800 mcg. To get the full 3 to 4 g of folic acid that are necessary for optimal health, you will need to take additional over-the-counter folic acid supplements or ask your doctor to prescribe a larger amount. For the purpose of making basic formulas less bulky, many manufacturers provide less than the minimum

TABLE 22.1

Basic Nutrition Vitamin/Mineral Formula

Vitanutrient	Daily Intake
Natural beta-carotene	3,000–6,000 IU
Vitamin A	1,500–3,000 IU
Vitamin B$_1$	30–60 mg
Vitamin B$_2$	24–48 mg
Niacin	15–30 mg
Niacinamide	30–60 mg
Pantothenic acid	75–150 mg
Pantethine	75–150 mg
Vitamin B$_6$	30–60 mg
Folic acid	2,000–4,000 mcg
Biotin	225–450 mcg
Vitamin B$_{12}$	180–240 mcg
Vitamin C	500–1,000 mg
Vitamin D$_2$	90–180 IU
Vitamin E	150–300 IU
Copper	600–1,200 mcg
Magnesium	50–100 mg
Calcium	200–400 mg
Choline	300–600 mg
Inositol	240–480 mg
PABA	300–600 mg
Manganese	12–24 mg
Zinc	24–48 mg
Citrus bioflavonoids	450–600 mg
Chromium	150–300 mcg
Selenium	120–240 mcg
N-acetyl-cysteine	60–120 mg
Molybdenum	30–60 mcg
Vanadyl sulfate	45–90 mcg
Octacosanol	450–900 mcg
Reduced glutathione	15–30 mg

requirement for calcium. If you select such a formula and your dietary calcium intake is low, you should include a 500-mg calcium tablet as part of your basic program. For best results, choose supplements made with calcium citrate or calcium lactate. Finally, when you select vitamin E supplements, choose only the natural kind.

In addition to your daily dose of vitamins and minerals, I recommend daily supplements of the essential fatty acids (refer back to Chapter 14 for details). The optimal dose is 400 mg each of borage oil (GLA), fish oil (EPA and DHA), and flaxseed oil (LNA), taken two to three times daily (for a total of 800 to 1,200 mg of each daily). Many manufacturers make a combined essential oils formula that contains all three forms.

Vitanutrient Solutions

The protocols that follow were created with the assumption that you are already taking the basic multivitamin/mineral formula outlined above. The vitanutrients in this basic formula are valuable for maintaining basic good health and helping to prevent many of the preventable diseases of aging. To augment your intake to reach the higher doses suggested in the protocols, subtract the amount of the vitanutrient in your daily formula from the larger amount in the protocol. The difference is the amount of the vitanutrient you need to add.

Space limitations restrict me to only the most important uses of vitanutrients for preventing and treating health problems, which follow.

Heart and Vascular Health

Antioxidants, from both diet and supplements, are extremely important for preventing heart disease and protecting your coronary arteries. You also need to maintain high levels of folic acid to remove artery-damaging homocysteine from your system. In addition to your basic vitamin/mineral formula, the vitanutrients in Table 22.2 are valuable for maximizing heart health. I've discussed many of them and their role in protecting your heart throughout this book.

TABLE 22.2

Vitanutrients for Heart and Vascular Health

Vitanutrient	Daily Intake
Magnesium	400–800 mg
Coenzyme Q_{10}	60–120 mg
L-carnitine	1,000–2,000 mg
Taurine	500–1,000 mg
Vitamin E	400–800 IU
Vitamin C	1,000–3,000 mg
Essential oils formula	3,600–7,200 mg
Mixed tocotrienols	100–200 mg
Chromium	200–400 mcg
Natural beta-carotene	25,000 IU
Ginkgo biloba	240–480 mg
B complex	50 mg
Folic acid	3–6 mg

High Cholesterol

As discussed in detail, your total cholesterol level alone is not a particularly accurate indicator of your risk of heart disease or stroke. A much better marker is your ratio of HDL cholesterol to triglycerides. In my experience there is rarely if ever a need for lipid-lowering drugs to reduce your LDL cholesterol, raise your HDL cholesterol, and improve your ratio of HDL to triglycerides. The vitanutrients in Table 22.3, in combination with a low-carbohydrate diet, should easily lower your total cholesterol. To be sure the program is helping you, you must work with your physician to monitor your blood lipid levels on a regular basis.

To help improve your ratio of triglycerides to HDL cholesterol, follow the high-cholesterol formula and add: carnitine, 1,500–3,000 mg; EPA/DHA from fish oil, 1,200–2,400 mg; chromium, 400–800 mcg; vanadyl sulfate, 15–30 mg.

TABLE 22.3

Vitanutrients for High Total Cholesterol

Vitanutrient	Daily Intake
Pantethine	600–1,200 mg
Inositol hexanicotinate	500–1,500 mg
Chromium	300–600 mcg
Essential oils formula	7,200 mg
Vitamin C	1,000–5,000 mg
Mixed fiber supplement	10 g
Lecithin granules	2–3 tbsp
Guggulipid	100–200 mg
Borage oil (GLA)	1,200–3,600 mg
Garlic	2,400–4,000 mg
Gamma oryzanol	300–600 mg
Mixed tocotrienols	200–400 mg
Natural beta-carotene	25,000–50,000 IU

High Blood Pressure

For many decades, elevated blood pressure was called "essential hypertension," which actually meant the cause was not known. All that has changed with a spate of research, led by Dr. Gerald Reaven of Stanford University, showing that most hypertension is caused by excessive insulin.

Dr. Reaven estimated that 60 percent of all hypertension patients have an exaggerated insulin response to dietary carbohydrates. At the Atkins Center, the dramatic lowering effect on the blood pressure of the low-carbohydrate, anti-insulin diet is seen in over 90 percent of our patients. The Atkins diet works well in combination with the vitanutrients listed in Table 22.4.

TABLE 22.4

Vitanutrients for Hypertension

Vitanutrient	Daily Intake
Taurine	1,500–3,000 mg
Magnesium	500–1,000 mg
Hawthorn	240–480 mg
Potassium aspartate	400–800 mg
Vitamin B$_6$	100–200 mg
Essential oils formula	3,600–7,200 mg
Garlic	2,400–3,200 mg
Coenzyme Q$_{10}$	100–200 mg
Carnitine	500–1,000 mg
Chromium	300–600 mcg

Blood Sugar Imbalances

As you surely appreciate by now, I believe that blood sugar imbalances are the most important nutrition-based diseases in the Western world—and they are becoming the most important in many developing parts of the world as well. The incidence of diabetes is exploding worldwide, with billions of new cases expected over the next few decades. Diabetes is a major disease in its own right and is also a major risk factor for coronary heart disease, stroke, kidney disease, and other serious complications. (For a thorough discussion of the entire issue of blood sugar, insulin, and the stages leading up to diabetes, refer back to Chapter 4.) Here I give two protocols. Table 22.5 lists vitanutrients that help keep the blood sugar in balance and ameliorate or prevent the early prediabetes stages and early type II diabetes. Table 22.6 is for prediabetics who need to bring elevated blood sugar down to normal levels and for type II diabetics who are now taking antidiabetes medications.

TABLE 22.5

Vitanutrients for Prediabetics

Vitanutrient	Daily Intake
Chromium	200–600 mcg
Zinc	50–100 mg
Magnesium	300–600 mg
Lipoic acid	150–300 mg
Coenzyme Q_{10}	45–90 mg
Biotin	2–4 mg
Essential oils formula	7,200 mg
Selenium	100–200 mcg
Vitamin B_6	75–150 mg

TABLE 22.6

Vitanutrients for Diabetics

Vitanutrient	Daily Intake
Chromium	500–1,000 mcg
Alphalipoic acid	300–600 mg
Vanadyl sulfate	30–60 mg
Coenzyme Q_{10}	90–180 mg
Biotin	7.5–15 mg
Inositol	800–1,600 mg
Zinc	90–180 mg
Niacinamide	30–600 mg
Magnesium	450–900 mg
Gymnema sylvestre	200–400 mg
Fenugreek	125–250 mg

Overweight and Obesity

Over half of all adult Americans are overweight and more than a quarter of all American children are overweight. In the long run this figure will translate into huge, extremely expensive amounts of poor health, lost productivity and pleasure in life, and early death.

Severe weight gain is actually a manifestation of insulin resistance, as discussed at length earlier. To counteract this tendency, I strongly recommend the strategy presented in *Dr. Atkins' New Diet Revolution*. This is the diet strategy that has worked for thousands of my patients and for the millions of people who bought my book and followed its advice. Diet alone, as I point out, will cause you to lose weight. When my low-carbohydrate, high-protein diet is combined with the vitanutrients in Table 22.7, however, blocked metabolic pathways are opened and weight loss is facilitated.

TABLE 22.7

Vitanutrients for Weight Loss

Vitanutrient	Daily Intake
Chromium	400–800 mcg
Carnitine	1,00–2,000 mg
Coenzyme Q_{10}	75–150 mg
Glutamine	2–4 grams
Phenylalanine	750–1,500 mg
Choline	750–1,500 mg
Inositol	1,000–2,000 mg
Methionine	400–800 mg
Lipoic acid	100–300 mg

Brain Nutrients

Keeping your cognitive abilities high is so important a part of your age-defying program that I devoted all of Chapter 18 to a discussion of vitanutrients that help. Table 22.8 gives you a beginning basic protocol.

TABLE 22.8

Brain Vitanutrients

Vitanutrient	Daily Intake
Thiamin	50–100 mg
Folic acid	3–6 mg
Phosphatidyl serine	200–400 mg
Phospatidyl choline	200–400 mg
Ginkgo biloba (standardized extract)	120–240 mg
Acetyl-l-carnitine	100–200 mg
Octacosanol	10–20 mg
Vitamin B_{12}	1,000–2,000 mcg
Vitamin B_6	30–60 mg

Menopause Symptoms

Contrary to the gospel as espoused by the medical establishment, the discomforts of menopause do not need to be treated with hormone replacement therapy. As I discussed in Chapter 13 on hormones, there are much safer alternatives with no side effects. Vitanutrients are extremely helpful at this time in a woman's life, when she needs optimal nutrition. As mentioned above, the large doses of folic acid recommended in Table 22.9 are best obtained with a doctor's prescription. However, women who need to shrink uterine fibroids, prevent breast cancer recurrences, or deal with endometriosis or fibrocystic breasts should keep supplemental folic acid below 600 mcg daily. The recommendations for pregnenolone and DHEA are

TABLE 22.9

Vitanutrients for Menopause Symptoms

Vitanutrient	Daily Intake
Folic acid	20–60 mg
Boron	6–18 mg
Pregnenolone	30–60 mg
DHEA	20–40 mg
Essential oils formula	3,600–7,200 mg
Vitamin E	400–1,200 IU
Vitamin B_6	150–300 mg
Gamma oryzanol	150–450 mg
B vitamin complex	50–100 mg
Chromium	200–600 mcg

based on the dosages most women need. As discussed in Chapter 13, however, you should work with your physician to determine your current blood levels and the amounts of vitanutrients that will restore your levels to those of a thirty-year-old.

Preventing and Treating Osteoporosis

Osteoporosis—thin, brittle bones that break easily—is a disease that is easily slowed or even prevented. A combination of exercise, natural hormones, and vitanutrients can be very helpful for dealing with this crippling disease. In general, the vitanutrients in Table 22.10, when combined with exercise, will help prevent and treat osteoporosis as well as do the powerful drugs that are commonly prescribed. When choosing a calcium supplement, select one made with calcium citrate or calcium

TABLE 22.10

Vitanutrients for Osteoporosis

Vitanutrient	Daily Intake
Folic acid	20–60 mg
Boron	6–12 mg
Calcium	800–1,600 mg
Vitamin D	400–800 IU
Magnesium	400–800 mg
Vitamin K	150–300 mcg
Silicon	100–300 mg
Lysine	500–1,000 mg
B vitamin complex	500–100 mg
Ipriflavone	300–600 mg

lactate for maximum absorption. Please refer back to the discussion of menopause symptoms in Chapter 13 for more information about folic acid and the hormones DHEA and pregnenolone.

Treating Inflammation

Inflammation is a general term for the swelling, redness, heat, and pain that usually accompany an injury or illness. A very common source of ongoing inflammation is arthritis—the affected joints swell and become painful. A standard medical treatment for arthritis is a nonsteroidal anti-inflammatory drug (NSAID) such as aspirin, ibuprofen, naproxen, and others. Even though many NSAIDs are now available over the counter, these medications can have serious side effects, such as intestinal bleeding. I much prefer to take a natural approach to inflammation and treat it with safe vitanutrients.

As discussed in Chapter 3, a more worrisome problem is inflammation of your blood vessels themselves, as indicated by the marker C-reactive protein (CRP). This can be very damaging to your heart. At the Atkins Center we are so concerned about CRP that we are constantly seeking new ways to treat it with vitanutrients and herbs. We have had good success with the formula listed in Table 22.11.

The vitanutrients in the table are those we now use for treating inflammation of all sorts. They are quite helpful, but this is an area where there is always room for improvement. We are currently studying the latest research and working with our patients to find new ways to relieve inflammation, particularly when CRP is the problem.

TABLE 22.11

Vitanutrients for Inflammation

Vitanutrient	Daily Intake
MSM (methyl sulfonyl methane)	1,500–3,000 mg
Essential oils formula	3,500–7,000 mg
Quercitin	800–1,600 mg
Turmeric	200–400 mg
Ginger	200–400 mg
Boswellia (standardized extract with 65% boswellic acid)	150–300 mg
Bromelain	400–800 mg
Bilberry	100–200 mg
Niacinamide	100–200 mg
Pantethine	100–200 mg
Vitamin C	1,000–2,000 mg

Prostate Protection

By the time a typical man reaches the age of sixty or so, he is quite likely to be experiencing the symptoms of benign enlargement of the prostate, also known as benign prostate hypertrophy (BPH). This condition, in which the prostate gland becomes swollen enough to obstruct urine flow, makes urination difficult and causes frequent trips to the bathroom during the night, interfering with restful sleep. This may actually cause a decline in your production in growth hormone, to say nothing of the tiredness the next day.

Standard medical treatment for BPH begins with strong drugs that often have unwanted side effects and proceeds to complication-laden, often unnecessary surgery that can leave the patient incontinent and impotent. The vitanutrient approach is far less harsh. The protocol in Table 22.12 is also excellent for supporting male reproductive health in general. You should plan on taking the supplements for at least three months before you notice a major improvement in your symptoms.

TABLE 22.12

Vitanutrients for Male Reproductive Health

Vitanutrient	Daily Intake
Saw palmetto (standardized extract)	250–500 mg
Pygeum africanum (standardized extract)	100–200 mg
Glutamic acid	50–1,000 mg
Glycine	250–500 mg
Alanine	250–500 mg
Manganese	20–40 mg
Essential oils formula	3,600–7,200 mg
Zinc	50–100 mg

23

Putting It All Together

The age-defying steps I've outlined in this book are designed to help you live a longer, healthier life. They're based on my years of clinical experience, combined with the latest cutting-edge research. There's nothing mysterious or difficult about my age-defying approach. The basic diet is easy to understand and even easier to follow. The vitanutrients I recommend and the other age-defying techniques I suggest are based on proven medicine and can be done by anyone. There's every reason to think that you too can benefit from them.

The world of age-defying research is very dynamic and exciting. In fact, it is so dynamic that your conventional physician may not be aware of the latest developments and may not understand all the age-defying techniques I've discussed. Any conscientious, knowledgeable, and open-minded physician should be able to work with you to achieve at least some of your age-defying goals. Here are some thoughts on how to go about it.

Working with Your Doctor

If, as I've talked about how to use laboratory tests to determine your blood lipids, insulin level, hormone levels, and more you thought to yourself, "I'm going to need a doctor to get the tests done," you were absolutely right. Only a physician can do the sort of testing you need and interpret the results for you, and only a physician can supervise some of the techniques I suggest.

To get the most from the age-defying concepts I've discussed, you not only need to know about the workings of your own body, you need to work with your doctor to verify that the changes you make in your diet, vitanutrient use, and lifestyle are having the desired effect.

Changing the World Of Health

I dedicated this book to my followers for a reason. I believe that what is really needed to transform today's medicine is a group of people who consider themselves my supporters, followers, adherents, or, as some people have called themselves, Atkids. Lest you think this is self-serving, please bear in mind that I have dedicated my life to making the world better for the people whose paths cross mine. What we need are people who can help change the medical establishment—a grassroots movement that ensures that the truth about health, instead of mainstream propaganda, gets out to everyone.

The most convincing argument we can deliver is our success in achieving the goal of this book: having a longer, healthier life span.

If you'd like to help effect the necessary changes in our society, I ask you to let us know who you are. Visit our interactive Web site at www.atkinscenter.com or call The Atkins Center at 001 212 7582110. We want to know how you are doing as you follow the age-defying diet revolution. Send us your case histories, your experiences, and your comments.

One Last Word

Today the breakthroughs in age-defying medicine come so frequently that I was adding information to this book until the absolute last possible moment. The cutting-edge research I discuss is the most up-to-date I could find. Yet in the short time it took to print this volume and get it into your hands, there doubtless will have been new scientific developments that could change your life for the better. As new developments arise in this fascinating area, I will be telling you about them on my Web site and in my newsletter, *Dr. Atkins' Health Revelations*.

Communication has been revolutionized by the Internet, so no longer does an author such as myself simply write a book and hope that people will read it and take its message to heart. Today the author and his readers can have a true interactive relationship. I welcome your comments and questions and look forward, with the help of my staff, to answering them. I hope you will be one of those people whose age-defying success serves as a role model for many more. That way, the movement toward making us all healthier, all more long-lived, will prevail.

APPENDIX

The Glycemic Index of Common Foods

The glycemic index measures the effect a particular food has on your blood sugar when you eat it. Foods that are high on the glycemic index raise your blood sugar higher than foods that are lower on the index. The standard against which foods are measured for the glycemic index is glucose, otherwise known as table sugar, which is given the rating 100. The glycemic index concept applies only to high-carbohydrate foods—foods that are high in protein or fat don't raise your blood sugar much if at all. The glycemic index is a useful tool for selecting foods for your age-defying diet—just look for foods that are as low on the index as possible. Bear in mind, however, that the index doesn't take into account factors that slow down how quickly a food raises your blood sugar. If you have some grapes (GI 45) for dessert after eating a high-protein meal, the fructose from the grapes will enter your system more slowly and thus raise your blood sugar more slowly as well.

The Glycemic Index

Food	Rating	Food	Rating
Maltose	110	Spaghetti	50
Glucose	100	Oatmeal	49
Baked potato	98	Grapes	45
Carrots	92	Orange	40
Honey	87	Apple	39
Cornflakes	80	Tomato	38
Whole wheat bread	72	Chickpeas	36
White rice	72	Lima beans	36
White bread	69	Yogurt	36
Shredded wheat	67	Whole milk	34
Brown rice	66	Pears	34
Raisins	64	Skim milk	32
Beets	64	Kidney beans	29
Bananas	62	Lentils	29
Corn	59	Grapefruit	26
Green peas	51	Plum	25
Potato chips	51	Cherries	23
Sweet potato	51	Peanuts	13

ENDNOTES

CHAPTER 1

1. U.S. Bureau of Census.
2. Castelli WP. Concerning the possibility of a nutritional . . . Arch Intern Med 1992; 152:1371–72.
3. Morbidity and Mortality Weekly Report 1999; 48:664–68.
4. Statistics from American Heart Association, based on National Heart, Long, and Blood Institute studies.
5. De Backer G et al. Lifetime-risk prediction: a complicated business. Lancet 1999; 353:82–83, 89–92.
6. Resource Utilization Among Congestive Heart Failure (REACH) Study statistics, March 1999; American Heart Association statistics, September 1999.

CHAPTER 2

1. Morbidity and Mortality Weekly Report 1999; 48:664–68.
2. Ibid.
3. Cohen AM, Fidel J, Cohen B et al. Diabetes, blood lipids, lipoproteins, and change of environment: restudy of the "new immigrant Yemenites" in Israel. Metabolism 1979; 28:716–28.
4. Al-Nuaim AR. Prevalence of glucose intolerance in urban and rural communities in Saudi Arabia. Diabet Med 1997; 14:595–602.
5. World Health Organization statistics; King H, Aubert RE, Herman WH. Global burden of diabetes, 1995-2025: prevalence, numerical estimates, and projections. Diabetes Care 1998; 21:1414–31.

CHAPTER 3

1. Stampfer MJ, Krauss RM, Ma J et al. A prospective study of triglyceride level, low-density lipoprotein particle diameter, and risk of myocardial infarction. JAMA 1996; 276:882-88.
2. Ibid.

3. Assmann G, Schulte H. The importance of triglycerides: results from the Prospective Cardiovascular Muenster (PROCAM) Study. Eur J Epidemiol 1992; Supplement 1:99–103; Assmann G, Schulte H. Relation of high-density lipoprotein cholesterol and triglycerides to incidence of atherosclerotic coronary artery disease (the PROCAM experience). Am J Cardiology 1992; 70:733–37.

4. Gaziano JM et al. Fasting triglycerides, high-density lipoprotein, and risk of myocardial infarction. Circulation 1997; 96:2520–25.

5. Reissel PK et al. Treatment of hypertriglyceridemia. Am J Clin Nutr 1966; 19:84–98.

6. Presentation by K Moysich, annual meeting International Society for Environmental Epidemiology, 7 September 1999.

7. Haim M, Benderly M, Brunner D et al. Elevated serum triglyceride levels and long-term mortality in patients with coronary heart disease: the Bezafibrate Infarction Prevention (BIP) Registry. Circulation 1999; 100: 475–82.

8. Bass KM, Newschaffer CJ, Klag MJ, Bush TL. Plasma lipoprotein levels as predictors of cardiovascular death in women. Arch Intern Med 1993; 153:2209–16.

9. Sanchez-Delgado E, Liechti H. Lifetime risk of developing coronary heart disease. Lancet 1999; 353:934.

10. Rath M, Pauling L. Immunological evidence for the accumulation of lipoprotein(a) in the atherosclerotic lesion of the hypoascorbemic guinea pig. Proc Natl Acad Sci USA 1990; 87:9388–90.

11. Fenech M. Towards promulgation of the healthy life span. Ann NY Acad Sci 1997; 854:23–36.

12. Graham IM, Daly LE, Refsum HM et al. Plasma homocysteine as a risk factor for vascular disease. The European Concerted Action Project. JAMA 1997; 277:1775–81.

13. Kark JD, Selhub J, Adler B et al. Nonlasting plasma total homocysteine level and mortality in middle-aged and elderly men and women in Jerusalem. Ann Intern Med 1999; 131:321–30.

14. American Heart Association recommendation. Homocysteine, Folic Acid and Cardiovascular Disease, 1998.

15. Internal Medicine News, 15 May 1999, 52.

16. Ridker PM, Cushman M, Stampfer MJ et al. Inflammation, aspirin, and the risk of cardiovascular disease in apparently healthy men. NEJM 1997; 336:973–79.

17. Ridker PM et al. Prospective study of C-reactive protein and the risk of future cardiovascular events among apparently healthy women. Circulation 1998; 98:731–33.

18. Ibid.

19. Ridker, Cushman, Stampfer et al. Inflammation, aspirin, and the risk of cardiovascular disease . . . [See Chap. 3, No.17]

20. Campbell LA, Kuo CC, Grayston JT. Chlamydia pneumoniae and cardiovascular disease. Emerging Infectious Diseases 1998; 4:571–79; Meier CR et al. Antibiotics and risk of subsequent first-time acute myocardial infarction. JAMA 1999; 281:427–31.

21. File TM, Bartlett JG, Cassell GH et al. The importance of Chlamydia pneumoniae as a pathogen: the 1996 consensus conference on Chlamydia pneumoniae infections. Infec Dis Clin Practice 1997; 6:S28–31.

22. National Heart, Lung, and Blood Institute statistics, August 1999.

23. Melnick JL et al. Cytomegalovirus antigen within human arterial smooth muscle cells. Lancet 1983; 2:644–47.

24. Melnick JL et al. Cytomegalovirus and atherosclerosis Eur Heart J 1993; supp. K:30–38.

CHAPTER 5

1. Perls TT, Silver MH. Living to 100. NY: Basic Books, 1998, 113.

2. Cerami A, Vlassare H, Brownlee M. Glucose and aging. Scientific American 1987; 256:90–96.

3. Diabetes Care 1999; 22:45–49.

4. Tominaga M, Fguchi H, Manaka H et al. Impaired glucose tolerance is a risk factor for cardiovascular disease, but not impaired fasting glucose: the Funagata diabetes study. Diabetes Care 1999; 22:920–24.

5. Smith MA et al. Advanced Maillard reaction end products are associated with Alzheimer disease pathology. Proc Nat Acad Sci USA 1994; 91:5710–14; Vitek MP et al. Advance glycation end products contribute to amyloidosis in Alzheimer disease. Proc Nat Acad Sci USA 1994; 91:4766–70.

6. Bucala R et al. Modification of low density lipoprotein by advanced glycation end products contributes to the dyslipidemia of diabetes and renal insufficiency. Proc Nat Acad Sci USA 1994; 91:9441–45.

7. Al-Abed Y et al. Inhibition of advanced glycation endproduct formation by acetaldehyde: role in the cardioprotective effect of ethanol. Proc Nat Acad Sci USA 1999; 96:2385–90.

8. Fournier AM, Gadia MT, Kubrusly DB et al. Blood pressure, insulin and glycemia in nondiabetic subjects. Am J Med 1983; 80:861–64.

9. Nestler JE, Beer NA, Jakubowicz J, Beer RM. Effects of a reduction in circulating insulin by metformin on serum dehydroepiandrosterone sulfate in nondiabetic men. J Clin Endocrinol Metab 1994; 78:549–54.

10. Buffington CK, Pourmotabbed G, Kitabchi AE. Case report: amelioration of insulin resistance in diabetes with dehydroepiandrosterone. Am J Med Sci 1993; 306:320–24.

11. Evans GW, Swensen G, Walters K. Chromium picolinate decreases calcium excretion and increases dehydroepiandrosterone (DHEA) in post menopausal women. FASEB J 1995; 9:A449.

CHAPTER 6

1. Harman D. Free radical theory of aging: role of free radicals in the origination and evolution of life, aging, and disease processes. In John JE Jr, Walford R, Harmon D et al., eds. Free Radicals, Aging and Degenerative Diseases. NY: Alan R. Liss, 1986, 3–49.

2. Harman D. The biological clock: the mitochondria? J Am Geriatrics Soc 1972; 20:145–47.

3. Diplock AT. Antioxidant nutrients and disease prevention. Am J Clin Nutr 1991, 53:189S–193S.

4. Harman D. Aging: minimizing free radical damage. Journal of Anti-aging Medicine 1999; 2:15–36.

5. Ibid.

CHAPTER 7

1. Weindruch R, Walford RL, Figiel S, Guthrie D. The retardation of aging in mice by dietary restriction: longevity, cancer, immunity and lifetime energy intake. J Nutr 1986; 116:641–54.

2. Walford R, Harris SB, Weindruch R. Dietary restriction and aging: historical phases, mechanisms, and current directions. J Nutr 1987; 117:1650–54.

3. Barzilai N, Gupta G. Revisiting the role of fat mass in the life extension induced by caloric restriction. J Gerontol A Biol Sci Med Sci 1999; 54:B89–98.

4. Manson, JE et al. Body weight and mortality among women. NEJM 1995; 333:677–87.

5. Bloom WL, Azar G et al. Comparison of metabolic changes in fasting obese and lean patients. Ann NY Acad Sci 1965; 131:623–31.

CHAPTER 8

1. Hodis HN, Mack WJ, LaBree L et al. Serial coronary angiographic evidence that antioxidant vitamin intake reduces progression of coronary artery atherosclerosis. JAMA 1995; 273:1849–54.

2. Comstock GW, Burke AE, Hoffman SC et al. Serum concentrations of alpha tocopherol, beta carotene, and retinol preceding the diagnosis of rheumatoid arthritis and systemic lupus erythematosus. Ann Rheum Dis 1997; 56:323–25.

3. Rimm EB, Stampfer MJ, Ascherio A et al. Vitamin E consumption and the risk of coronary heart disease in men. NEJM 1993; 328:1450–56.

4. Stampfer MJ, Hennekens CH, Manson JE et al. Vitamin E consumption and the risk of coronary disease in women. NEJM 1993; 328:1444–49.

5. Stephens NG, Parsons A, Schofield PM et al. Randomised controlled study of vitamin E in patients with coronary disease: Cambridge Heart Antioxidant Study (CHAOS). Lancet 1996; 347:781–86.

6. Kushi LH, Folsom AR, Prineas RJ et al. Dietary antioxidant vitamins and death from coronary heart disease in postmenopausal women. NEJM 1996; 334:1156–62.

7. Nyssonone K, Parviainen MT, Salonen R et al. Vitamin C deficiency and risk of myocardial infarction: prospective population study of men from eastern Finland. BMJ 1997; 314:634–38.

8. Johnston CS, Thompson LL. Vitamin C status of an outpatient population. J Am Coll Nutr 1998; 17:366–70.

9. Vita JA et al. Low plasma ascorbic acid predicts the presence of an unstable coronary syndrome. J Am Coll Cardiology 1998; 31:980–86.

10. Podmore ID, Griffiths HR, Herbert KE et al. Vitamin C exhibits pro-oxidant properties. Nature 1998: 392:6676.

11. Duthie SJ, Ma A, Ross MA, Collins AR. Antioxidant supplementation decreases oxidative DNA damage in human lymphocytes. Cancer Res 1996 56:1291–95.

12. Suadicani P, Hein HO, Gyntelberg F. Serum selenium concentration and risk of ischaemic heart disease in a prospective cohort study of 3000 males. Atherosclerosis 1992; 96:33–42.

13. Paleologos M, Cuming RG, Lazarus R. Cohort study of vitamin C intake and cognitive impairment. Am J Epidemiology 1998; 148:45–50.

14. Schmidt R. Plasma antioxidants and cognitive performance in middle-aged and older adults: results of the Austrian Stroke Prevention Study. J Am Geriatrics Soc 1998; 46:1407–10.

15. Sano M, Ernesto C, Thomas RC, Klauber MR et al. A controlled trial of selegiline, alpha-tocopherol, or both as a treatment for Alzheimer's disease: the Alzheimer's disease cooperative study. NEJM 1997; 336:1216–22.

16. Ziegler D, Hanefeld M, Ruhnau KJ et al. Treatment of symptomatic diabetic peripheral neuropathy with the anti-oxidant alpha-lipoic acid: a 3-week multicenter randomized controlled trial (ALADIN Study). Diabetologica 1995; 38:1425–33.

17. Henson DE, Block G, Levine M. Ascorbic acid: biologic functions and relation to cancer. J Natl Cancer Institute 1991; 83:547–50.

18. Block G. Vitamin C and reduced mortality. Epidemiology 1992; 3:189–91.

19. Heinonen OP, Albanes D, Virtamo J et al. Prostate cancer and supplementation with alpha-tocopherol and beta-carotene: incidence and mortality in a controlled trial. J Natl Cancer Institute 1998; 90:440–46.

20. Clark LC et al. Effect of selenium supplementation for cancer prevention with carcinoma of the skin: a randomized controlled trial. JAMA 1996; 276:1957–63.

21. Colditz GA. Selenium and cancer prevention: promising results indicate further trials required. JAMA 1996; 276:1985.

22. Yoshizawa K, Willett WC, Morris SJ et al. Study of prediagnostic selenium level in toenails and the risk of advanced prostate cancer. J Natl Cancer Institute 1998; 90:1219–24.

23. Leske MC, Chylack LT Jr, He Q et al. Antioxidant vitamins and nuclear opacity: the longitudinal study of cataract. Ophthalmology 1998; 105:831–36.

24. Seddon JM, Christen WG, Manson JE et al. The use of vitamin supplements and the risk of cataract among U.S. male physicians. Am J Pub Health 1994; 84:788–92.

25. Jacques PF, Taylor A, Hankinson SE et al. Long-term vitamin C supplement use and prevalence of early age-related lens opacities. Am J Clin Nutr 1997; 66:911–16.

26. Bendich A, Langseth L. The health effects of vitamin C supplementation: a review. J Am Coll Nutr 1995; 14:124–36.

CHAPTER 9

1. Schnohr P, Thomsen OO, Riis Hansen P et al. Egg consumption and high-density-lipoprotein cholesterol. Journal of Internal Medicine 1994; 235:249–51.

2. Hu FB, Stampfer M, Rimm EB et al. A prospective study of egg consumption and risk of cardiovascular disease in men and women. JAMA 1999; 281:1387–94.

3. Beyer RE. The participation of coenzyme Q in free radical production and antioxidation. Free Radic Biol Med 1990; 8:545–65; Lenaz G, Battino M, Castelluccio C et al. Studies on the role of ubiquinone in the control of the mitochondrial respiratory chain. Free Radical Research Communications 1990; 8:317–27.

4. Crane FL, Navas P. The diversity of coenzyme Q function. Mol Aspects Med 1997; 18:S1–6.

5. Esterbauer H, Striegl G, Puhl H, Rotheneder M. Continuous monitoring of in vitro oxidation of human low density lipoprotein. Free Radical Research Communications 1989; 6:67–75.

6. Reiter RJ. Oxygen radical detoxification process during aging: the functional importance of melatonin. Aging (Milano) 1995; 5:340–51.

7. Poeggeler B, Reiter RJ, Tan DX et al. Melatonin, hydroxyl radical-mediated oxidative damage, and aging: a hypothesis. J Pineal Res 1993; 14:151–68.

8. Reiter RJ, Guerrero JM, Garcia JJ, Acuña-Castroviejo D. Reactive oxygen intermediates, molecular damage, and aging. Relation to melatonin. Ann NY Acad Sci 1998; 854:410–24.

9. Brezinski A. Melatonin in humans. NEJM 1997; 336:186–95.

10. Ibid.

CHAPTER 10

1. Beecher GR, Khackik F. Qualitative relationship of dietary and plasma carotenoids in human beings. Ann NY Acad Sci 1992; 669:320–21.

2. Ford ES, Will JC, Bowman BA, Narayan KM. Diabetes mellitus and serum carotenoids: findings from the Third National Health and Nutrition Examination Survey. Am J Epidemiology 1999; 149:168–76.

3. Sies H, Stahl W. Vitamins E and C, beta-carotene, and other carotenoids as antioxidants. Am J Clin Nutr 1995; 62:1315S–21S.

4. Bendich A, Olson JA. Biological action of carotenoids. FASEB Journal 1989; 3:1927–32.

5. Gester H. Potential role of beta-carotene in the prevention of cardiovascular disease. International Journal of Vitamin and Nutrition Research 1991; 61:277–91.

6. Klipstein-Grobusch K, Geleijnse JM, den Breeijen JH et al. Dietary antioxidants and risk of myocardial infarction in the elderly: the Rotterdam Study. Am J Clin Nutr 1999: 69:261–66.

7. Hennekens CH, Buring JE, Manson JE et al. Lack of effect of long-term supplementation with beta-carotene on the incidence of malignant neoplasms and cardiovascular disease. NEJM 1996; 334:1145–90.

8. Diplock AT. Safety of antioxidant vitamins and beta-carotene. Am J Clin Nutr 1995; 62:1510S–16S.

9. Omenn GS, Goodman GE, Thornquist MD et al. Effects of a combination of beta carotene and vitamin A on lung cancer and cardiovascular disease. NEJM 1996; 334:1150–55.

10. Van Poppel G, Goldbohm RA. Epidemiological evidence for beta carotene and cancer prevention. Am J Clin Nutr 1995; 62:1393S–402S.

11. Jumaan AO, Holmberg L, Zack M et al. Beta-carotene intake and risk of postmenopausal breast cancer. Epidemiology 1999; 10:49–53.

12. Presentation by M Stampfer, American Society of Clinical Oncology annual meeting, Denver, 19 May 1997.

13. Acevedo P, Bertram JS. Liarozole potentiates the cancer chemopreventive activity of and the upregulation of gap junction communication and connexin 43 expression by retinoic acid and beta-carotene in 10T1/2 cells. Carcinogenesis 1995; 16:2215–22.

14. Nieper H. Technology, Medicine, and Society. MIT Verlag 1985, 268–69.

15. Santos MS et al. Beta-carotene-induced enhancement of natural killer cell activity in elderly men: an investigation of the role of cytokines. Am J Clin Nutr 1998; 68:164–70.

16. Canfield LM, Forage JW, Valenzuela JG. Carotenoids as cellular antioxidants. Proceedings of the Society of Experimental Biology and Medicine 1992; 200:260–65.

17. Di Mascio P, Kiaser S, Sies H. Lycopene as the most efficient biological carotenoid singlet oxygen quencher. Arch Biochem Biophys 1989; 274:532–38.

18. Giovannucci E, Ascherio A, Rimm EB, Stampfer MJ et al. Intake of

carotenoids and retinol in relation to risk of prostate cancer. J Natl Cancer Institute 1995; 87:1767–76.

19. Presentation by O Kucuk, Karmanos Cancer Institute, American Association for Cancer Research meeting, 12 April 1999.

20. Giovannucci E. Tomatoes, tomato-based products, lycopene, and cancer: review of the epidemiological literature. J Natl Cancer Institute 1999; 91:317–31.

21. Garcia-Closas R, Agudo A, Gonzales CA, Riboli RE. Intake of specific carotenoids and flavonoids and the risk of lung cancer in women in Barcelona, Spain. Nutr Cancer 1998; 32:154–58.

22. Kohlmeier L, Kark JD et al. Lycopene and myocardial infarction risk in the EURAMIC Study. Am J Epidemiology 1997; 146:618–26.

23. Riso P, Pinder A et al. Does tomato consumption effectively increase the resistance of lymphocyte DNA to oxidative damage? Am J Clin Nutr 1999; 69:712–18.

24. Christen WG, Glynn RJ et al. A prospective study of cigarette smoking and the risk of age-related macular degeneration in men. JAMA 1996; 276:1147–51; Seddon, JM, Willett WC et al. A prospective study of cigarette smoking and the risk of age-related macular degeneration in women. JAMA 1996: 276:1141–46.

25. Snodderly DM. Evidence for protection against age-related macular degeneration by carotenoids and antioxidant vitamins. Am J Clin Nutr 1995; 62S:1448S–61S.

26. Seddon JM, Ajani UA, Perduto RD et al. Dietary carotenoids, vitamins A, C, and E, and advanced age-related macular degeneration. JAMA 1994; 272:1413–20.

27. Sommerburg O et al. Fruits and vegetables that are sources for lutein and zeaxanthin: the macular pigment in human eyes. Brit J Ophthalmology 1998; 83:907–10.

28. Seddon, Ajani, Perduto et al. Dietary carotenoids . . . [See No. 26 above]

29. Stampfer MJ, Willett WC. Olestra and the FDA. NEJM 1996; 335:669.

CHAPTER 11

1. Prior RL, Cao G. Antioxidant capacity and polyphenolic components of teas: implications for altering in vivo antioxidant status. Proc Soc Exp Biol Med 1999; 220:255–61.

2. Gao YT, McLaughlin JK, Blot WJ et al. Reduced risk of esophageal cancer associated with green tea consumption. J Natl Cancer Institute 1994; 85:855–58.

3. Katiyar SK, Mukhtar H. Tea in chemoprevention of cancer: epidemiologic and experimental studies. International J of Oncology 1996; 8:221–38.

4. Ahmad N, Feyes DK et al. Green tea constituent epigallocatechin-3-

gallate and induction of apoptosis and cell cycle arrest in human carcinoma cells. J Natl Cancer Institute 1997; 89:1881–86.

5. Presentation by DJ Morré and DM Morré, American Society for Cell Biology annual meeting, December 1998.

6. Luo M, Kannar K. Wahlqvist ML, O'Brien RC. Inhibition of LDL oxidation by green tea extract. Lancet 1997; 349:360–61.

7. Sesso HD et al. Coffee and tea intake and risk of myocardial infarction. Am J Epidemiology 1999; 149:162–67.

8. Keli SO et al. Dietary flavonoids, antioxidant vitamins, and incidence of stroke: the Zutphen Study. Archives Intern Med 1996; 156:637–42.

9. Haqqi TM et al. Prevention of collagen-induced arthritis in mice by a polyphenic fraction from green tea. Proc Natl Acad Sci USA 1999; 96:4524–29.

10. Yam TS, Hamilton-Miller JM, Shah S. The effect of a component of tea (Camellia sinensis) on methicillin resistance, PBP2' synthesis, and beta-lactamase production in Staphylococcus aureus. Journal of Antimicrobial Chemotherapy 1998; 42:211–16.

11. Ioky K et al. Antioxidative activity of quercetin and quercetin monoglucosides in solution and phospholipid bilayers. Biochem Biophys Acta 1995; 1234:99–104.

12. Breithaupt-Groegler K, Ling M, Boudoulas H, Betz GG. Protective effect of chronic garlic intake on elastic properties of aorta in the elderly. Circulation 1997; 96:2649–55.

13. Kosceilny J, Kluessendorf D, Latza R et al. The antiatherosclerotic effect of Allium sativum. Atherosclerosis 1999; 144:237–49.

14. Science News 19 April 1997; 151:239.

15. Witte JS et al. Relation of vegetable, fruit, and grain consumption to colorectal adenomatous polyps. Am J Epidemiology 1996; 144:1015–25.

CHAPTER 12

1. Barrett-Connor E, Goodman-Gruen D. The epidemiology of DHEAS and cardiovascular disease. Ann NY Acad Sci 1995; 774:259–70.

2. Morales AJ, Nolan JJ, Nelson JC, Yen SS. Effects of replacement dose of dehydroepiandrosterone in men and women of advancing age. J Clin Endocrinology 1994; 78:1360–67.

3. Barrett-Connor E, Khaw KT, Yen SS. A prospective study of dehydroepiandrosterone sulfate, mortality, and cardiovascular disease. NEJM 1986; 315:1519–24.

4. Newcomer LM, Manson JE, Barbieri RL et al. Dehydroepidandrosterone sulfate and the risk of myocardial infarction in US male physicians: a prospective study. Am J Epidemiology 1994; 140:870–75; Herrington DM. Dehydroepiandrosterone and coronary atherosclerosis. Ann NY Acad Sci 1995; 774:271–80.

5. Herrington. Dehydroepiandrosterone and coronary atherosclerosis. Ann NY Acad Sci 1995; 774:271–80.

6. Khorram O, Vu L, Yen SS. Activation of immune function by dehydroepiandrosterone (DHEA) in age-advanced men. Journal of Gerontology 1997; 52:1–7.

7. Gordon GB, Helzlsouer KJ, Comstock GW. Serum levels of dehydroepiandrosterone and its sulfate and the risk of developing bladder cancer. Cancer Res 1991; 51:1366–69; Schwartz AG, Pashko LL. Mechanism of cancer preventive action of DHEA. Ann NY Acad Sci 1995; 774:180–86.

8. Yen SS, Morales AJ, Khorram O. Replacement of DHEA in aging men and women. Ann NY Acad Sci 1995; 774:128–42.

9. Roberts E. Pregnenolone from Selye to Alzheimer and a model of the pregnenolone binding site on the GABA receptor. Biochemical Pharmacology 1995; 49:1–16.

CHAPTER 13

1. Barrett-Connor EL. Testosterone and risk factors for cardiovascular disease in men. Diabetes Metab 1995; 21:156–61.

2. Krotkiewski M, Bjorntorp P. The effect of progesterone and of insulin administration on regional adipose tissue cellularity in the rat. Acta Physiol Scand 1976; 96:122–27.

3. Beck P, Eaton RP, Arnett DM et al. Effect of contraceptive steroids on arginine-stimulated glucagon and insulin secretion in women: I-Lipid physiology. Metabolism 1975; 24:1055–65.

4. Hulley S, Grady D, Bush T et al. Randomized trial of estrogen plus progestin for secondary prevention of coronary heart disease in postmenopausal women: Heart and Estrogen/progestin Replacement Study (HERS) Research Group. JAMA 1998; 280:605–13.

5. Lee JR. Is natural progesterone the missing link in osteoporosis prevention and treatment? Medical Hypotheses 1991; 35:316–18.

6. Agnusdei D, Bufalino L. Efficacy of ipriflavone in established osteoporosis and long-term safety. Calcif Tissue Int 1997; 61:S23–27; Agnusdei D, Crepaldi G, Isaia G et al. A double blind, placebo-controlled trial of ipriflavone for prevention of postmenopausal spinal bone loss. Calcif Tissue Int 1997; 61:142–47.

7. Rosen T, Johannsson G et al. Consequences of growth hormone deficiency in adults and the benefits and risks of recombinant human growth hormone treatment. A review paper. Horm Res 1995; 43:93–99.

8. Mantzoros CS et al. Insulin resistance: the clinical spectrum. Adv Endocrinol and Metab 1995; 259:1703–05.

9. Iranmanesh A, Lizarralde B, Veldhuis JD. Age and relative adiposity are specific negative determinants of the frequency and amplitude of growth hormone (GH) secretory bursts and the half-life of endogenous GH in healthy men. J Clin Endocrinol Metab 1991; 73:1081–88.

10. Rudman D et al. Effect of human growth hormones in men over 60 years old. NEJM 1990; 323:1–6.

11. Fazio S et al. A preliminary study of growth hormone in the treatment of dilated cardiomyopathy. NEJM 1996; 334:809–14.

12. Moses AC. Recombinant human insulin-like growth factor 1 increases insulin sensitivity and improves glycemic control in type II diabetes. Diabetes 1996; 45:91–100.

13. Bennett RM, Clark SC, Walczyk J. A randomized double-blind placebo-controlled study of growth hormone in the treatment of fibromyalgia. Am J Med 1998; 104:227–31.

14. Waters D et al. Recombinant human growth hormone, insulin-like growth factor 1, and combination therapy in AIDS-associated wasting. Ann Intern Med 1996; 125:865–72.

15. Thompson RL. J Clin Endocrinol Metab 1998; 83:M77–84.

16. Yen SS, Morales AJ, Khorram O. Replacement of DHEA in aging men and women. Potential remedial effects. Ann NY Acad Sci 1995; 774:128–42.

17. Alba-Roth J, Muller OA, Schopohl J et al. Arginine stimulates growth hormone secretion by suppressing endogenous somatostatin secretion. J Clin Endocrinol Metab 1988; 67:1186–89.

18. Borst JE et al. Studies of GH secretogogues in man. J Am Geriatrics Soc 1995; 42:532–34.

19. Corpas E, Blackman MR, Roberson R et al. Oral arginine-lysine does not increase growth hormone or insulin-like growth factor 1 in old men. J Gerontology 1993; 48:M128–33.

20. Welbourne T. Increased plasma bicarbonate and growth hormone after oral glutamine load. Am J Clin Nutr 1995; 61:1058–61.

21. Rolandi E et al. Changes of pituitary secretion after long-term treatment with Hydergine, in elderly patients. Acta Endocrinologica 983; 102:32–36.

CHAPTER 14

1. Castelli. Concerning the possibility of a nutritional . . . [See Chap. 1, Note No. 2]

2. Corr LA, Oliver MF. The low fat/low cholesterol diet is ineffective. Eur Heart J 1997; 18:18–22.

3. Ravnskov U. The questionable role of saturated and polyunsaturated fatty acids in cardiovascular disease. J Clin Epidemiol 1998; 51:442–60.

4. Presentation by DL Tirshwell, 24th Annual AHA Conference on Stroke and Cerebral Circulation, 10 February 1999.

5. Bang HO, Dyerberg J, Hjorne N. The composition of food consumed by Greenland Eskimos. Acta Med Scand 1976; 200:69–73.

6. Burr MI, et al. Effects of changes in fat, fish, and fibre intakes on death and myocardial reinfarction: diet and reinfarction trial (DART). Lancet 1989; 2:757–61.

7. Albert CM, Hennekens CH, O'Donnell CJ et al. Fish consumption and risk of sudden cardiac death. JAMA 1998; 279:23–28.

8. Fernandez E, Chatenoud L, La Vecchia C et al. Fish consumption and cancer risk. Am J Clinical Nutr 1999; 70:85–90.

9. Belluzi A, Brignola C, Campieri M et al. Effect of an enteric-coated fish-oil preparation on relapses in Crohn's disease. NEJM 1996; 334:1557–60.

10. Watkin BA, Seifert MF, Allen KG. Importance of dietary fat in modulating PGE2 responses and influence of vitamin E on bone morphometry. Word Rev Nutr Diet 1997; 82:250–59.

11. Stoll AL, Severus WE, Freeman MP et al. Omega 3 fatty acids in bipolar disorder: a preliminary double-blind, placebo-controlled trial. Archives of General Psychiatry 1999; 56:401–12.

12. Zurier RB, Rosetti RG, Jacobson EW et al. Gamma-linolenic acid treatment of rheumatoid arthritis. A randomized, placebo-controlled trial. Arthritis Rheum 1996; 39:1808–17.

13. Hu FB, Stampfer MJ, Manson JE et al. Dietary intake of alpha-linolenic acid and risk of fatal ischemic heart disease among women. Am J Clin Nutr 1999; 69:890–97.

14. Hansen JC, Pedersen HS, Mulvad G. Fatty acids and antioxidants in the Inuit diet. Arctic Med Res 1994; 53:4–17.

15. Hu FB, Stampfer MJ, Manson JE et al. Frequent nut consumption and risk of coronary heart disease in women: prospective cohort study. BMJ 1998; 317:1341–45.

16. Solfrizzi V, Panza F, Torres F et al. High monounsaturated fatty acids intake protects against age-related cognitive decline. Neurology 1999; 52:1563–69.

17. Willett WC, Stampfer MJ, Manson JE et al. Intake of trans fatty acids of risk of coronary heart disease among women. Lancet 1993; 341:581–85.

18. Mann GV. Metabolic consequences of dietary trans fatty acids. Lancet 1994; 343:1268–71.

19. Barnard DE, Sampugna J, Berlin E et al. Dietary trans fatty acids modulate erythrocyte membrane fatty acyl composition and insulin binding in monkeys. J Nutr Biochem 1990; 1:190–95; Kuller LH. Trans fatty acids and dieting [letter]. Lancet 1993; 341:1093–94.

20. Ascherio A, Katan MB, Stampfer MJ. Trans fatty acids and coronary heart disease. NEJM 1999; 340:1994–98.

21. Enig MG. Trans Fatty Acids in the Food Supply. Silver Spring, MD: Enig Associates, 1993.

CHAPTER 15

1. Bernstein J et al. Depression of lymphocyte transformation following oral glucose ingestion. Am J Clin Nutr 1977; 30:613.

2. Canfield LM, Forage JW, Valanzuela JG. Carotenoids as cellular antioxidants. Proceedings of the Society of Experimental Biology and Medicine 1992; 200:260–65.

3. Santos MS, Meydani SN, Leka L et al. Natural killer cell activity in

elderly men is enhanced by beta-carotene supplementation. Am J Clin Nutr 1996; 64:772–77.

4. Chasen-Taber L et al. J Am Coll Nutr 1996; 15:136–43.

5. Bendich A. Food Technology 1987; 41:112–14.

6. Hemila H, Herman ZS. Vitamin C and the common cold: a retrospective analysis of Chalmer's review. J Amer Coll Nutr 1995; 14:116–23.

7. Henson DE, Block G, Levine M. Ascorbic acid: biologic functions and relation to cancer. J Natl Cancer Institute 1991; 83:547–50.

8. Block, G. Vitamin C and reduced mortality. Epidemiology 1992; 3:189–91.

9. Meydani SN, Meydani M, Blumberg JB et al. Vitamin E supplementation and in vivo immune response in healthy elderly subjects: a randomized controlled trial. JAMA 1997; 277:1380–86.

10. Watson RR, Benedict J, Mayberry JC et al. Supplementation of vitamins C and E and cellular immune function in young and aging men. Ann NY Acad Sci 1990; 498:530–33.

11. Ford ES, Sowell A. Serum alpha-tocopherol status in the United States population: findings from the Third National Health and Nutrition Examination Survey. Am J Epidemiology 1999; 150:290–300.

12. Mossad SB, Macknin ML et al. Zinc gluconate lozenges for treating the common cold. Ann Internal Med 1996; 125:81–88.

13. National Center for Health Statistics data from NHANES III.

14. Fortes C et al. The effect of zinc and vitamin A supplementation on immune response in an older population. J Am Geriatrics Soc 1998; 46:19–26.

15. Corti MC et al. Serum iron level, coronary artery disease, and all-cause mortality in older men and women. Am J Cardiology 1997; 79:120–27.

16. Scaglione F, Cattaneo G, Alessandria M, Cogo R. Efficacy and safety of the standardized ginseng extract G 115 for potentiating vaccination against common cold and/or influenza syndrome. Drugs under Experimental and Clinical Research 1996; 22:65–72.

17. See DM, Broumand N, Sahl L, Tilles JG. In vitro effects of echinacea and ginseng on natural killer and antibody-dependent cell cytotoxicity in healthy subjects and chronic fatigue or acquired immunodeficiency syndrome patients. Immunopharmacology 1997; 35:229–35.

18. Song Z et al. Ginseng treatment reduces bacterial load and lung pathology in chronic Pseudomonas aeruginosa pneumonia in rats. Antimicrobial Agents and Chemotherapy 1997; 41:961–64.

19. Zhang et al. Ginseng extract scavenges hydroxyl radical and protects unsaturated fatty acids from decomposition caused by iron-mediated lipid peroxidation. Free Radical Biology and Medicine 1996; 20:145–50.

20. Jensen GL et al. A double-blind, prospective, randomized study of glutamine-enriched compared with standard peptide-based feeding in critically ill patients. Am J Clin Nutr 1996; 64:615–21.

21. Caroleo M, Frasca D, Nistico G et al. Melatonin as immunomodulator in immunodeficient mice. Immunopharmacology 1992; 23:81–89.

CHAPTER 16

1. Herzenberg M. Scandinavian Journal of Rheumatology 1995; 24:207–11.

2. Lancet 1992; 239:1263–64.

3. Staessen JA, Roels HA, Emelianov D et al. Environmental exposure to cadmium, forearm bone density, and risk of fractures: prospective population study. Lancet 1999; 353:1140–44.

4. Lin JL, Ho HH, Yu CC. Chelation therapy for patients with elevated body lead burden and progressive renal insufficiency. Ann Internal Med 1999; 130:7–13.

5. Rudolph CJ, McDonagh EW, Wussow DG. The effect of intravenous ethylene diamine tetraacetic acid (EDTA) upon bone density levels. J Advancement Med 1988; 1:79.

6. Deucher DP. EDTA chelation therapy: an antioxidant strategy. J Advancement Med 1988; 1:182.

7. Kindness G, Frackelton JP. Effect of ethylene diamine tetraacetic acid (EDTA) on platelet aggregation in human blood. J Advancement Med 1989: 2:519.

8. World Health Organization. Environmental Health Criteria for Inorganic Mercury, 118. Geneva: WHO, 1991.

9. Frustaci A, Magnavita N, Chimenti C et al. Marked elevation of myocardial trace elements in idiopathic dilated cardiomyopathy compared with secondary cardiac dysfunction. J Am Coll Cardiology 1999; 33:1578–83.

CHAPTER 17

1. Grundy SM, Balady GJ et al. Primary prevention of coronary heart disease. Circulation 1998; 97:1876–87.

2. Hakim AA, Curb JD et al. Effects of walking on coronary heart disease in elderly men: the Honolulu Heart Program. Circulation 1999; 100:9–13.

3. Ekelund LG et al. Physical fitness as a predictor of cardiovascular mortality in asymptomatic North American men. NEJM 1988; 319:1379–84.

4. Wei M, Gibbons LW, Mitchell TL et al. The association between cardiorespiratory fitness and impaired fasting glucose and type 2 diabetes mellitus in men. Ann Internal Med 1999; 130:89–96.

5. Thune I, Brenn T et al. Physical activity and the risk of breast cancer. NEJM 1997; 336:1269–75; Tang R, Wang JY, Lo SK, Hsieh LL. Physical activity, water intake and risk of colorectal cancer in Taiwan: a hospital-based case-control study. International Journal of Cancer 1999; 82:484–89.

6. Leveille SG, Guralnik JM et al. Aging successfully until death in old age: opportunities for increasing active life expectancy. Am J Epidemiology 1999; 149:654–64.

7. Ferrucci L, Izmirlian G et al. Smoking, physical activity, and active life expectancy. Am J Epidemiology 1999; 149:645–53.

8. Fiatarone MA, Marks EC et al. High-intensity strength training in nonagenarians: effects on skeletal muscle. JAMA 1990; 263:3029–34.

9. Jette AM et al. Exercise—it's never too late: the strong-for-life program. Am J Pub Health 1999; 89:66–72.

10. Hayashi T, Tsumura K, Suematsu C et al. Walking to work and the risk of hypertension in men: the Osaka Health Survey. Ann Internal Med 1999; 130:21–26.

11. Hakim AA, Curb JD, Petrovitch H et al. Effects of walking on coronary heart disease in elderly men: the Honolulu Heart Program. Circulation 1999; 100:9–13.

12. Manson JE, Hu FB et al. A prospective study of walking as compared with vigorous exercise in the prevention of coronary heart disease in women. NEJM 1999; 341:650–58.

13. Kramer AF, Hahn S, Cohen NJ et al. Ageing, fitness and neurocognitive function. Nature 1999; 400:418–19.

14. Shore S, Shinkai S et al. Immune responses to training: how critical is training volume? J Sports Med Phys Fitness 1999; 39:1–11.

15. Presentation by JT Venkatramen, 4th International Society for Exercise and Immunology Symposium, May 1999.

CHAPTER 18

1. Vitek MP, Bhattacharya K, Glendening JM et al. Advanced glycation end products contribute to amyloidosis in Alzheimer disease. Proc Natl Acad Sci USA 1994; 91:4766–70.

2. Ross GW, Petrovitch H et al. Characterization of risk factors for vascular dementia: the Honolulu-Asia Aging Study. Neurology 1999; 53:337–43.

3. Coffey CE, Saxton JA, Ratcliff G et al. Relation of education to brain size in normal aging: implications for the reserve hypothesis. Neurology 1999; 53:189–96.

4. Bassuk SS, Glass TA, Berkman LF. Social disengagement and incident cognitive decline in community-dwelling elderly persons. Ann Internal Med 1999; 131:165–73.

5. Hopfenmuller W. Proof of the therapeutical effectiveness of a ginkgo biloba special extract: meta-analysis of 11 clinical trials in aged patients with cerebral insufficiency. Arzneim-Forsch 1994; 1005–13; Maurer K. Clinical efficacy of Ginkgo biloba special extract Egb 761 in dementia of the Alzheimer type. J of Psych Research 1997; 31:645–55.

6. Le Bars PL, Katz MM et al. A placebo-controlled, double-blind, randomized trial of an extract of ginkgo biloba for dementia. JAMA 1997; 278:1327–32.

7. Crook T et al. Effects of phosphatidylserine in age-associated memory impairment. Neurology 1991; 41:644–49.

8. Monteleone P, Beinat L, Tanzillo C et al. Effects of phosphatidyl serine on the neuroendocrine response to physical stress in humans. Neuroendocrinology 1990; 52:243–48.

9. Pettegrew JW et al. Clinical and neurochemical effects of acetyl-l-carnitine in Alzheimer's disease. Neurobiology of Aging 1995; 16:1–4; Salvioli G, Neri M. L-acetylcarnitine treatment of mental decline in the elderly. Drugs in Experimental Clinical Research 1994; 20:169–76.

10. Flood JF, Morley JF, Roberts E. Pregnenolone sulfate enhances post-training memory processes when injected in very low doses into limbic system structures. Proc Natl Acad Sci 1995; 92:10806–10.

11. Ibid.

12. Lindenbaum J, Rosenberg IH, Wilson PW et al. Prevalence of cobalamin deficiency in the Framingham elderly population. Am J Clinical Nutrition 1994; 60:2–11.

13. Clarke R, Smith D, Jobst KA et al. Folate, vitamin B12, and serum total homocysteine levels in confirmed Alzheimer disease. Arch Neurol 1998; 55:1449–55.

14. Morrison LD, Smith DD, Kish SJ. Brain S-adenosylmethionine levels are severely decreased in Alzheimer's disease. Journal of Neurochemistry 1996; 67:1328–31.

CHAPTER 21

1. NHANES III survey statistic from CDC's National Center for Health Statistics.

2. National Heart, Lung, and Blood Institute statistics.

3. Cao G, Sofic E, Prior RL. Antioxidant capacity of tea and common vegetables. J Agric Food Chem 1996; 44:3426–31; Wang H, Cao G, Prior RL. Total antioxidant capacity of fruits. J Agric Food Chem 1996; 44:701–05.

4. Steinmetz KA, Potter JD. Vegetables, fruit, and cancer prevention: a review. J Am Diet Assoc 1996; 96:1027–39.

5. Bobak M et al. An ecological study of determinants of coronary heart disease rates: a comparison of Czech, Bavarian and Israeli men. Int J Epidemiol 1999; 28:437–44.

6. Cao G, Booth SL, Sadowski JA, Prior RL. Increases in human plasma antioxidant capacity after consumption of controlled diets high in fruit and vegetables. Am J Clin Nutr 1998; 68:1081–87.

7. Cao G, Russel RM, Lischner N, Prior RL. Serum antioxidant capacity is increased by consumption of strawberries, spinach, red wine or vitamin C in elderly women. J Nutr 1998; 128:2382–90.

INDEX

ℐtart Defying Your Age Today!

Eat well and stay young! Dr. Atkins, using 30 years of experience with nutrition and the latest scientific breakthroughs, has created a new Age-Defying Diet. Using this simple program you can . . . defy your age!

If you enjoyed reading *Dr Atkins' Age-Defying Diet Revolution* and would like to learn more, you might also want to read:

- *Dr. Atkins' New Diet Revolution* (Revised and Updated)
  The #1 best selling book that started it all! Includes new chapters and information about this revolutionary weight loss program.
  Available from Vermilion. To order by mail in the UK, telephone Bookpost on 01624 677237.

- *Dr. Atkins' Quick & Easy New Diet Cookbook*
  Mouthwatering recipes that go from stovetop to tabletop in 30 minutes or less.

ℋow to Learn More About the Atkins Center

Established in 1970, the Atkins Center for Complementary Medicine is an eighty-staff, six-story medical facility in the heart of New York City. The Atkins Center's mission is to first address major health disorders through vitanutrient therapies, diet modifications, and lifestyle changes that can enhance the body's own restorative powers before patients resort to prescription drugs and/or surgical procedures. More than sixty thousand patients have been treated at the Atkins Center for a wide variety of disorders, including cancer, arthritis, asthma, diabetes, heart/cardiovascular disease, chronic fatigue, multiple sclerosis, as well as weight problems.

For further information on the Atkins Center, please call (001) 212 758 2110.

Visit us on the web at www.atkinscenter.com